Lydia W Stephens

Heart Problems

Lydia W Stephens

Heart Problems

ISBN/EAN: 9783742813817

Manufactured in Europe, USA, Canada, Australia, Japa

Cover: Foto ©Lupo / pixelio.de

Manufactured and distributed by brebook publishing software (www.brebook.com)

Lydia W Stephens

Heart Problems

Heart Problems.

BY

LYDIA W. STEPHENS.

"I were content, could I be but a flower
Up at the foot of those."
T. BUCHANAN READ.

PHILADELPHIA:
DAUGHADAY & BECKER,
424 WALNUT STREET.
1870.

Entered according to Act of Congress, in the year 1869, by
LYDIA W. STEPHENS,
In the Clerk's Office of the District Court of the United States, in and for the Eastern District of Pennsylvania.

TO

MY DEAR UNCLE AND FORMER GUARDIAN,

JOSEPH DAVIS,

AS A

TOKEN OF SINCERE GRATITUDE

FOR HIS UNTIRING AND DISINTERESTED KINDNESS

TO THE

ORPHAN AND THE MOTHERLESS,

I MOST AFFECTIONATELY

DEDICATE THIS VOLUME.

Norristown, Pa.

PREFACE.

HAVE solved them all—all these intricate problems—as one by one the unfolding of the pages of Life's Volume has revealed them to me. Difficult has been the solution, and mournful the result of some. Yet, with a grateful heart, I now review them, conscious that to me has been justly awarded that common lot of humanity, to enjoy, to suffer, and endure.

Heart-problems! Who has not solved them? Who has not felt the ecstatic joy, or the overwhelming grief, which their solution brings? And who does not hope, one day, to present them to the Great Teacher, in the humble confidence that the same omniscience that has discerned every conflict between the weak flesh and the willing spirit, will pronounce upon them the welcome plaudit of "well-done?"

The oft-repeated solicitations of personal friends have eventually induced me to subject this volume of my original productions to public criticism. Many of them have heretofore appeared in some of the periodicals of my own and sister States—mostly over a fictitious signature—while others have, until now, retained their manuscript form. Some of them were written previous to the dark hours of the rebellion; others, during its most appalling tragedies; and yet others, since the last four years of a nominal peace have enabled us to partially recover from the murderous assaults upon our national existence.

To the advocates of non-resistance who may peruse this volume, a portion of its contents may seem like apologies for, if not eulogiums of the barbarous practice of settling, by means of a wholesale human carnage, whatever difficulties may arise between nations. Yet, such was by no means the spirit which prompted those productions. War, with its horrid accompaniments, has always been hateful to me. I loathe its very name. But, a war waged for the emancipation of a long-oppressed people, and participated in by the truest type of American manhood, was a theme calculated to awaken the deepest sympathy, and furnish inspiration for the humblest pen. I admire, almost reverence, that truly Christian spirit that resists not evil; yet when, contrasting the homes of those which the war had death-dreared, with the few that had escaped that desolation—I have asked myself the question, Which of these is bearing the heaviest cross?—every feeling of justice and humanity has prompted me to a decision in favor of the former. And when, too, in those days of sorest trial, I have seen friends and connexions dissuading their loved ones from obeying what had seemed to them the voice of duty—their country's call—and, in a short time, beheld those same loved ones cold in death, either from disease or accident, I have been led to exclaim—Surely, the hand of God is in this thing! and they who refuse to make sacrifice to their nation, in this, her hour of peril, may be called upon to make greater sacrifices, in a moment when they deem themselves most secure therefrom. Hence, whether a pacific or a warlike spirit pervades these effusions, one motive only has prompted their production—that of keeping forever paramount the great principles of truth, justice, and humanity.

The book, with whatever merits or demerits it may possess, is now alike at the mercy of sympathizing friends and a scrutinizing public, and its Authoress, while she asks for it a fair and impartial criticism, claims the privilege of advancing in its behalf this one brief argument—
" 'Tis the heart gives value to words."

L. W. S.

CONTENTS.

	PAGE.
PREFACE,	5
INQUIRE WITHIN,	13
THE SPIRIT BRIDE,	18
GO AND DO THOU LIKEWISE,	30
AUTUMNAL MUSINGS,	32
THE OLD CHESTNUT TREE,	34
LET ME DIE AT HOME,	37
SEARCH THE SCRIPTURES,	40
THE THUNDER STORM,	43
PERPETUAL BLOOM,	46
HOLD ON!	48
THEY SLUMBER HERE,	50
HOME THOUGHTS,	54
OUR SUNBEAM,	57
OUR SHADOW,	59
THE ROOM WHERE LOVED ONES DIE,	61
HEAVENLY TREASURES,	63
LET JEHOVAH JUDGE!	65
CAST THY BREAD UPON THE WATERS,	67
DYING EMBERS,	69
LANDSCAPES OF LIFE,	71
HOW SHALL WE KNOW THEM THERE?	76
'TIS HOME WHERE THE HEART IS,	79

CONTENTS.

	PAGE.
WITHOUT AN ENEMY,	84
THE FROST UPON THE PANE,	87
REMINISCENCES,	90
THE CHILD'S MATIN HYMN,	93
GONE TO REST,	96
DESCRIPTION OF A WINTER MORNING,	98
MY VOCATION,	101
LUCK AND PLUCK,	103
I WOULDN'T BE JEALOUS IF I WERE YOU,	105
CHILDHOOD'S HOME,	107
BIRTH-DAY PENCILLINGS,	110
SUMMER CLOUDS,	113
TO MY NIECE, ON HER NINTH BIRTH-DAY,	115
"GILPIN'S ROCKS."—CECIL COUNTY, MARYLAND,	118
AUTUMN LEAVES,	120
THE SPIRIT LAND,	122
GOD MADE US TO BE HAPPY,	124
FUGITIVE LAYS,	126
CURLING SMOKE,	129
FIDELITY,	131
COME UP HIGHER,	133
RIPPLES IN THE GRAIN,	138
GONE BEFORE,	141
CHARITY,	144
THE OLD HOMESTEAD,	147
SUMMER FRIENDS,	150
FAITHFUL IS HE THAT CALLETH YOU,	154
THE THREE SOLILOQUIES,	156
GOD TEMPERS THE WIND TO THE SHORN LAMB,	160
UNDER-CURRENTS,	162
IMPROMPTU TO WATER,	165
TO THE SCHUYLKILL RIVER,	169
PRACTISE WHAT YOU PREACH; OR, EXAMPLE BETTER THAN PRECEPT,	172
OMNISCIENCE,	175
RANDOM THOUGHTS,	177

CONTENTS.

	PAGE
THE INEBRIATE'S WIFE,	180
MY OTHER SELF,	183
OUR FATHER!	186
THE WRECK OF A BROKEN LIFE,	188
WHITE SWEARING,	191
INDEPENDENCE MUST HAVE LIMITS,	193
THE EXODUS OF THE NINETEENTH CENTURY,	195
IN MEMORIAM,	198
AFTER THE BATTLE,	200
NAVIS REPUBLICÆ,	203
WHEN THE WAR ENDS,	206
FORT PILLOW,	209
OUR DEAD HEROES,	212
WHAT I SAW, HEARD, AND THOUGHT, ETC.,	216
FROM GETTYSBURG,	225
STRENGTH THROUGH ADVERSITY,	227
NOT RETURNED,	236
OUR NATION'S GRIEF,	240
IMMORTALS,	245
OUR ENSIGN,	253
GATHERED TO HIS FATHERS,	257
ONE YEAR IN THE SPIRIT-LAND,	260
GOING TO THE SPRINGS,	262
EARTH'S GREAT ONES,	267
THE SIGHING OF THE PINES,	269
IT IS FINISHED,	272

INQUIRE WITHIN.

STANZAS SUGGESTED BY SOME OF THE STIRRING EVENTS
OF THE WINTER OF 1859-60.

WITHIN this age of humbug and pretence,
When men of nonsense pass for men of sense;
When so-called teachers pompously profess
A tact and talent which they don't possess;
When shrewd attorneys, claiming what they please,
Enrich their purses from their clients' fees;
When would-be doctors swell their patients' bills,
By puffing "sovereign balms" and "cure-all pills;"
When Pharisaic cavillers at sin
Steal Heaven's garb "to serve the devil in;"
When worldly-wise, manœuvering mammas
Would fain entrap young gents with rich papas;

When wily politicians hourly seek
Lucrative offices both fat and sleek;
And *principle*—that guardian of the free—
Is sacrificed for *popularity;*
'Tis mete that all Life's duties who begin,
Should first this motto learn—INQUIRE WITHIN.

Pray note our Congress halls this present term!
Of wide dissensions the well-nourished germ:
Our periodicals, with vain regret,
Each day and hour proclaim, " No Speaker Yet!"
While Greeley, as his *Tribune* circulates,
In witty language, it denominates
A place in which our learned men of state
Have met to carry on a brisk debate.
The "Black Republicans" at once agree
No one but Sherman shall their speaker be;
While Southerners with scorn and terror look
On all who would encourage "Helper's Book."
Some slander'd representatives would fain
Newspaper paragraphs at length explain;
From Stevens' tongue sarcastic arrows fly;
And Hickman moves adjournment, *sine die!*
What is the matter? Such delay is sin!
Why don't some cooler heads inquire within?

INQUIRE WITHIN.

Now pause we where imposing walls arise,
And spire points upward to th' arching skies.
Come, let us enter—everywhere we see
The evidence of pride and pageantry;
Seeming to bear unto the startled ear,
The heartless words—" *No poor may enter here !*"
The organ sounds—Christ's messenger has come,
His mission is to lead earth's wand'rers home.
In prayer he kneels—the strains of music cease,
He seeks to break the bread of life and peace.
List to his words! Can you among them trace
Ideas suited to his hearers' case?
Ah, no! too frequently they're gilded o'er,
To screen the crimes his soul would else deplore!
Sin's sinfulness his spirit's eye can't see;
'Tis dazzled by his glittering salary.
Thus God's own courts are made the courts of sin,
Because His tenants don't inquire within.

Anon my muse the social circle gains;
Where Fashion proud her regal sway maintains;
She leads me through those richly garnished halls,
Thronging with gentry making "New Year's calls;"
She bids me mark that swarthy Cuban king
His costly gifts to yon fair lady bring!

Bids me a " Diamond Wedding" to behold!
Whose guests, arrayed in satins, pearls, and gold,
Now issue forth from that imposing dome,
Of wealth and luxury the princely home.
They pass in state along the crowded street;
The great cathedral door at length they greet;
They enter, and in solemn language take
Those holy vows which Death alone should break.
To moralize my muse would now begin:
I wonder if they both inquire within.

Lo! near Potomac's shore we next are seen,
Where Harper's Ferry opes a fearful scene;
Hark! from her arsenal the clash of arms
Grows fiercer, louder, as the contest warms.
What means it?—List! A small, undaunted band,
Possessed of an idea great and grand,
Obedient to their honor'd Chieftain's word,
" Commissioned," as he terms it, " from the Lord,"
Fired with the zeal that bought *our* liberty,
Another race from thraldom seek to free.
" Madman! Fanatic!" is the phrenzied cry:
" Martyr!" resounds in solemn symphony,
As he, the truthful, brave, doth calmly come
Forth from his cell to meet a felon's doom.

Let us not marvel, if, across the main,
Such news arouse a Hugo's just disdain !
Virginia, 'tis to thee we owe this scene !
Pause then, and honestly inquire within !

And now, kind friends, my humble task is done ;
No laurels have I gained, no trophies won ;
But, if I have amid this uncouth rhyme,
Devoid of language, graceful or sublime,
Awakened in some warmly throbbing heart
A new resolve to act the better part,
Distrust appearance, shun deception's car,
And learn to view Life's objects as they are ;
To join with fearless soul the moral fight,
And don the badge of justice, truth, and right ;
To seek, with heart sincere, that grace so free,
Christ deigns to offer unto you and me ;
If this be done, my purpose is attained,
My wishes have been met, my object gained.
Then may we, when our sovereign Judge shall look
To our accounts within His mystic Book,
Present a page, unblemished by a sin,
To Him whose searching eye inquire within.

THE SPIRIT BRIDE.

ONCE, within the dewy summer, shaded by a sighing grove,
Sat and chatted three young maidens, telling o'er their tales of love.
In her turn a witching fairy—zephyrs toying with her curls,
Clad in vestments light and airy, answered—" Now I tell you, girls,
If I thought I'd never marry, 'twould to me be source of dread;
For of all the hateful creatures none excel a prim old maid;
Stiffly starched, and cross, and fretful, ugly as they well can be,
Never loved and never loving—from such fate deliver me!"

Thus outspoke the bright-eyed Cora—Cora Lynn,
    the village pet;
Then, reproving, Maud Magregor raised to her her
    eyes of jet,
Saying, "You've forgotten, surely, in the bold ha-
    rangue you've made,
That our loving, loved Aunt Rosie is herself 'a prim
    old maid,'
Happy with her foster-children in her cottage by the
    sea—
She'll at least prove one exception, Cora, to your
    theory."
"Aunt Rosalbert, I'd forgotten," Cora blushingly
    replied.
"But come, girls, let's seek her cottage by the briny
    Ocean's side!
Somehow I now feel romantic; and, perchance, if e'er
    she loved,
She will tell us all the story, how her faith was tried
    and proved."
At her cottage door Aunt Rosie welcomed them with
    friendly smile,
Gave them seats beneath the woodbine, gaily chat-
    ting all the while;
But, when they make known their errand, transient
    clouds that smile efface,

Just as summer clouds at noonday flit across the
    sun's bright face.
Gaining then her wonted calmness, thus the kindly
    spinster spoke,
Words, whose earnest, deep-toned utt'rance slumber-
    ing chords of mem'ry woke:
"To begin aright my story, I my audience must
    bear
Unto my dear home of childhood, when I knew not
    grief or care;
To a home hard by our cottage, where, in olden
    luxury,
Dwelt a wealthy Irish noble, with his wife and chil-
    dren three;
Two were grown almost to girlhood; one, a brave
    and handsome boy,
Who, though seven years my senior, was my child-
    hood's pride and joy;
Charmed by Nature's rustic beauties roamed we
    through the woodlands wild—
He a tall and graceful stripling, I a frail and slender
    child.
Soon I knew my first great sorrow—death our happy
    threshold crossed;—
Placed two names upon the record of my early loved
    and lost.

Then that wealthy Irish noble kindly, thoughtfully did come,
Proffering my dying parents their lone orphan child a home.
Faithfully he kept that promise, faithfully and fondly too;
And my foster-mother, sisters, nought but fondness ever knew.
Soon those loving foster-sisters breathed, in accents soft and low,
Hymen's nuptials at the altar—left us other homes to know;
While the noble son and brother, earnest, talented, and brave,
To the lonely one beside him kind attention ever gave;
Little dreaming that such kindness might, in some unguarded hour,
Chain each ardent aspiration by Love's ever-conquering power;
Little dreaming that the praises given by others all the while,
Caused no pleasure, if those virtues won from him no answering smile.
But 'twas mine soon to discover—though against its power I strove—

While I loved him fondly, wildly, his was but a
 brother's love;
For, one night, 'mid Fashion's mazes, we a graceful
 beauty view,
With the mingled rose and lily clust'ring 'round her
 eyes of blue.
Soon I saw my earthly idol seek that beauteous
 being's side;
Then each hope I'd vainly cherished slowly in my
 bosom died;
For I knew that such a being would that idol's
 homage claim,
And forsake her home parental to assume his
 honored name.
When he led her to the altar, rousing all my woman's
 pride,
Calmly I performed each duty of the bridesmaid to
 the bride;
Nor was aught deceitful mingled even with an act
 like this;
For her fate with his was blending, and her happiness was his;
But I learned how much of torture human bosoms
 can conceal,
While in secret they are mourning sorrows they dare
 not reveal.

THE SPIRIT BRIDE.

When the festal throng was over sought I solitude's
retreat;
Pouring out my heartfelt anguish humbly at my
Saviour's feet.
There I found that consolation which none ever seek
in vain,
And with spirit chastened, strengthened, took life's
burden up again;
From my neck removed the necklace, tore the gar-
land from my brow,
Feeling that such costly trifles only mocked my
spirit now.
Arthur's home was bright as sunlight, children clus-
ter'd 'round his hearth;
Till the lovely one who bore them, fading slowly—
passed from earth;
Then, unto his death-dreared household earnestly he
bade me come,
For my honored foster-parents late had sought
another home.
Bade me once again his life-path with my presence
deign to bless;—
Comforting the lone, bereaved—fostering the motherless.
For a while I hesitated—shrinking from the world's
cold sneers—

But the urgent voice of duty overcame all other fears.
Entered on my new-found life-path, tranquil happiness was mine,
Though I worshipped, still unheeded, at my dearest earthly shrine.
Scarce a twelvemonth yet was numbered in the records of the past,
Ere again o'er Arthur's threshold dire disease relentless passed:
His once firm, elastic footstep feebler grew from day to day,
And I now, with keenest sorrow, marked him slowly fade away.
Once, while sadly o'er him watching, struggling with my soul's unrest,
He in tones both faint and faltering, thus my listening ear addressed :—
'Darling Rose, my Rose, mavourneen, listen to my accents now,
While you wipe, with hand caressing, clammy sweats from off my brow.
I am dying, Rose, mavourneen—slowly, feebly comes my breath,
And e'en now I feel the dampness of the chilling vale of death;

And I'd fain to you, mavourneen, my heart's history reveal,
Ere the sepulchre's closed portals all that history conceal.
I would speak of one, mavourneen, one who loved me fondly, well;
Gone from earth in youth and beauty with the countless host to dwell;—
I would speak of her, mavourneen, tell you of my spirit's thrall
Since I, in a thoughtless moment, utter'd words I'd now recall.
Dazzled by Kate's matchless beauty—lured by her enticing charms,
Once I fancied that I loved her—woo'd and won her to my arms;
But that day-dream scarce had faded ere your girlish form arose,
Moving like a shade between us in my spirit's deep repose.
Brief the love that Kate awakened—yours was lasting as my life;
Ere our marriage-vows were plighted felt I this internal strife;
But I never yet had spoken, Rosa, of my love to you,

And the seal remained unbroken; honor bade me thus to do;
And you seemed so calm, unmoved, at my dazzling bridal scene,
That I felt all unreturned would my love to you have been.
But, since you became an inmate of my desolated home,
Since Disease upon my vitals with his ravages has come,
Since so anxiously you've watched me with a fervor nought could pall,
I have learned your painful secret—Rosa, now I know it all.
Yes, I know it—long have known it—and to tell you felt no dread;
But respect was due, mavourneen, to the memory of the dead.
Sharing wholly my affections, as she thought, confidingly,
She has passed from earth to heaven—to our home beyond the sky.
Happy now among the angels doth her ransom'd spirit dwell,
While to you, my first and only loved one, I this story tell.

Be a mother to my children! Love, protect them as
 your own!
Keeping sacred still the mem'ry of the parents they
 have known!
And, though here you have not trodden in Love's
 pathway by my side,
None may doubt your claims in heaven; for you are
 my spirit-bride.'
Thus he lived and thus departed—he, my early, only
 love—
And he now awaits my coming in celestial bliss
 above.
Yonder come his merry children bounding through
 the wicket gate,
From their walk upon the sea-beach—Carl, Rosal-
 bert, Blanche, and Kate."
"But, Aunt Rosie," now responded frank, outspoken
 Effie Nohr,
"Had you ne'er another suitor?" "Yes, my darling,
 many more!
I with Arthur sought those mazes where I frequent-
 ly would meet
Those who cast in rich profusion Cupid's off'rings at
 my feet.
Charms I had—so flatt'rers told me—charms, accom
 plishments were mine,

While my ample fortune brought me wily suitors to
    my shrine,
But, when hearts like mine, so constant, so unchang-
    ing in their love,
Once have centered their affections, nought can those
    affections move."
  As the summer sun, reclining gently on his
    crimson bed,
Seemed to seek repose from labor, homeward they
    their journey sped.
Chastened by Aunt Rosie's story, wiser for the truth
    it taught,
Praying for a heart as constant each that night her
    chamber sought.
  Years have flown since that bright ev'ning, and
    upon each youthful brow
Care has lightly left her traces; two are sober
    matrons now;
But the third—the bright-eyed Cora—Cora Lynn,
    the village pet—
Reader, could you, would you think it?—Cora is not
    married yet!
Vainly friends and kindred rally—nothing can her
    purpose move,

As she laughingly informs them she'll not marry till
    she loves;
For Aunt Rosie's simple story long ago removed the
    dread
Pictur'd in her girlish fancy of the epithet—old
    maid.

GO AND DO THOU LIKEWISE!

THOUGHTS SUGGESTED WHILE LISTENING TO AN ORATION ENTITLED "THE MORAL HERO," DELIVERED IN FULTON HALL, LANCASTER, PA., BY ONE OF THE GRADUATES OF FRANKLIN AND MARSHALL COLLEGE, IN THE SUMMER OF 1859.

In one of Lancaster's capacious halls,
   That proudly bears immortal Fulton's name,
I sat and listened to the echoing fall
   Of footsteps treading in the path to fame.

Footsteps of those who proudly came to bear
   The trophies which their arduous toil had won;
Those fadeless laurels on their brows to wear,
   That tell of noble actions, nobly done.

I listened, too, to music's stirring notes,
   Borne in rich melody upon the air;
While strains of eloquence alternate float
   In manly tones from those assembled there.

GO AND DO THOU LIKEWISE.

And there was one—a slender, dark-eyed youth,
    Of pleasing, frank address, and earnest mien;
Forth from whose lips pure gems of sterling truth
    Flash'd like bright rays shed from Sol's glitt'ring sheen.

His theme—" The Moral Hero "—noble theme
    For orator's harangue or author's pen;
His words all potent and enchanting seem,
    Portraying duty to his fellow-men.

He spoke of those who, in the cause of truth,
    Come boldly forth to battle for the right;
And urged on all, alike in age or youth,
    To don, in proud array, Truth's armor bright.

My unknown friend, though I no more may see
    Thy form, nor listen to thy earnest tone;
May'st *thou*, in ages of futurity,
    In Truth's great cause blush not to stand alone.

Earth needs such moral heroes—Go thou forth!
    And what thou preachest strive to practise too!
God aid thee in a cause so fraught with worth,
    And bless thy actions, earnest, just and true!

AUTUMNAL MUSINGS.

There's a landscape, lovely and serene,
    That I from my chamber view;
I've admired it oft in the summer time,
    And now th' autumnal hue,
Spread o'er each tree, and plant, and flower,
    Portrays a richer scene,
Than when Nature smiled her loving smiles,
    Arrayed in robes of green.

Far in the distance waves a wood,
    While nearer we behold
Proud, undulating, fertile fields,
    Of purest, richest mould.
Some, autumn's sober robes have donn'd;
    While some in verdure glow;
Like to a ray of hope upon
    Submission's placid brow.

AUTUMNAL MUSINGS.

I know not why, but these autumn days
   Make me sadder now than wont,
And phantom forms of perished joys
   My soul's deep recess haunt.
I used to love their drap'ry rich,
   And joy in their gorgeous dies;
As they hung like richest tapestry
   'Neath an Indian Summer's skies.

For I knew that summer again would come,
   With em'rald robes so bright;
And we'd all forget the robes she wore
   'Neath th' hoar frost's icy blight.
She will come again to some, I know,
   But it may not be to me;
And the solemn thoughts that pervade my soul
   A warning of this may be.

Hast ordained it thus, omniscient One?
   Shall my life-cord soon be riven?
Then let Thy sov'reign will be done
   On earth as it is in heaven!
Yet ere in its eternal home
   My soul shall with rapture glow,
Mayst Thou, great Censor, approving scan
   My mission fulfill'd below!

THE OLD CHESTNUT-TREE.

STANZAS INSCRIBED TO MY FRIENDS AT WOOD LAWN, MONTGOMERY COUNTY, PA.

When first I knew thee, ancient tree,
Like to an islet in the sea
   Thou stoodst all alone;
Swaying thy sturdy banches there,
Freely within th' ambient air,
As sways his sceptre some proud heir
   Unto a regal throne.

Time passed; and in the years agone,
Upon thy verdant, sloping lawn,
   A habitation 'rose;
Then, in their turn, exotics grew;
With care transplanted for their hue
Of emerald, retained through
   Stern winter's storms and snows.

THE OLD CHESTNUT-TREE.

Yet all unconscious thou hast stood—
Proud relic of the ancient wood
  Of our immortal Penn;
Unconscious of thy rivals 'round,
In silent majesty profound,
Peerless, undaunted still, thou'rt found
  Among the haunts of men.

And well thou mayst—in thee we see
Both beauty and utility
  Judiciously combined;
The Schuylkill, laving at thy base,
Fills not more faithfully its place,
Uniting sturdy strength with grace,
  To benefit mankind.

Though oft we see thee brown and sere,
Grave sentinel, an object dear
  To me thou'st e'er been known;
Warm hearts are beating 'neath thy shade.
Warm hearts and true; and there have played
Children whose little lives have shed
  Bright sunshine o'er my own.

Long may the loved ones clustered there,
And kept by the protecting care

THE OLD CHESTNUT-TREE.

Of a blest Hand divine,
As many joys and pleasures know
Within their constant breasts to glow,
And ever in their life-path flow,
   As they have strewn on mine.

And long may'st thou, my aged friend,
With arms still seeming to extend
   A welcome unto me,
And all who to thy shades are drawn,
As in the halcyon days agone,
Stand, monarch of that wooded lawn—
   Time-honored chestnut-tree.

LET ME DIE AT HOME.

Some say that the fittest time to die
  Is, when fading leaves are strewn
In beauty 'neath the arching sky,
  By the gusts of Autumn blown;
But I care not whether Spring flowers gay,
  Or Summer's blossoms bloom
Around the freshly-moulded clay,
  That forms my new-made tomb.
I care not whether th' Autumn's blast,
  Or th' angry Winter storm,
Shall moan above the narrow house
  That holds my clay-cold form.
I only ask, when relentless Death
  With his fatal dart shall come,
And bid me yield my fleeting breath,
  That I may die at home.

For sure 'twould be sweeter far to die
    With loved ones 'round my bed;
Where the glistening tear in affection's eye,
    In silent grief is shed.
Where a true friend's hand shall press my brow,
    Or a familiar form
Shall mark my struggling spirit bow
    Before Death's gathering storm;
Where my last, faltering accents fall
    On each attentive ear,
And the words I breathe are heard by all
    Who will hold their mem'ry dear.
Ah, yes! methinks at whatever hour
    Death's mandate sure might come,
'Twould lessen its o'erwhelming power,
    If I could die at home.

When my freed soul shall wing its way
    To the mansions of the blest,
I would not have the stranger pray
    For that soul's eternal rest.
I would not have the stranger heap
    The clods above my grave—
Such a tomb may serve for those who sleep
    Like th' patriot warrior brave.

But when within its narrow bed
  My lifeless form is laid,
Let friendship's gentle tears be shed—
  By her hands let my grave be made.
God grant that whatever my fate may be,
  'Mid whatever scenes I roam,
When my soul shall pass to eternity,
  That I may die at home.

SEARCH THE SCRIPTURES.

"Search the Scriptures; for in them ye think ye have eternal life: And they are they which testify of me."—John v. 39.

Yes, search them through ! if ye would know
    The gems of holy truth,
Revealed upon each sacred page
    To guide the path of youth;
Or of the comfort which they give
    To the desponding soul,
When sorrow's overwhelming waves,
    Upon our pathway roll.

Ages have passed since God to man
    This precious volume gave;
Designed to show the wondrous plan,
    From sin our race to save;
And oft the skeptic proud has dar'd
    Its records to deny,
And spoken scornfully of all
    The truths that in it lie.

But as the diamond, which, conceal'd
    Far from each solar ray,
More brightly shines when 'tis reveal'd
    Amid the light of day;
So truth, though falsely crushed to earth
    By proud, presuming men,
Rises with more intrinsic worth
    Unto her sphere again.

And Christ, the Holy, and the Just,
    The Saviour of mankind,
When veiled in mortal flesh below,
    Their value thus defined :—
"Employ them not in useless strife!
    But search them through!" said he;
"In them ye have eternal life;
    They testify of me."

Of Him, the meek and lowly One,
    The Son and Sent of God;
Who, for the sins of all mankind,
    This vale of sorrow trod;
What nobler theme to contemplate,
    E'en for the worldly-wise,
Than Him, the Almighty Potentate,
    The Sov'reign of the Skies?

None! and sublimer, purer thoughts,
　　You'll seek in vain to find,
Than are within this holy Book
　　Profusedly combined!
Then search them through! for unto us
　　This treasure has been given,
To guide our wayward, wand'ring souls
　　Into the gates of Heaven.

THE THUNDER STORM.

Lo! from yon low'ring ebon cloud
   Comes forth the lightning's gleam!
While Thunder's notes reverberate
   O'er valley, hill, and stream.

Near and more near the clouds approach,
   More stunning is the sound;
While patt'ring rain-drops thickly fall,
   Like glittering pearls around.

I love to gaze on scenes like this,
   Scenes so sublime and grand;
And mark the skill and power divine
   Of an Almighty hand.

But why, within the doubting heart,
   Do fears so oft arise,
When viewing grandeur like to this,
   Within the raging skies?

THE THUNDER STORM.

'Tis true that danger seems more near
   In such an hour as this;
And proves to man there reigns above,
   A Power more great than his.

But yet, that overruling Power
   Protection can bestow,
The same amid the storm or calm,
   On mortals here below.

We're ever at His mercy plac'd,
   He guards each vessel frail;
Whether the sunlight gems life's waves,
   Or rudest winds assail.

The storm has ceased! Upon yon cloud
   The rainbow bright appears!
And we amid these calmer scenes
   Forget our recent fears!

Father! Oh, help us all to feel,
   In ev'ry stage of life,
Thy awful power, as when we mark
   Thy elements in strife!

And guide our actions, that we may
  'Mid all the storms of earth,
Look forth in faith to see Thee place
  Thy " bow of promise " forth!

PERPETUAL BLOOM.

THOUGHTS ON SEEING A ROSE-TREE BLOOMING DURING A SNOW STORM.

I saw it blooming 'mid the snow;
   Each bright and beauteous bud,
So fair and fragile in its form,
   The howling blast withstood;
And seemed to smile, calm and serene,
   Although the low'ring cloud
Had veiled its taper leaves of green
   Beneath a snowy shroud.

And as I gazed, I thought—how like
   Life's landscape this appears;
When ceaseless bloom Hope's blossoms bright,
   'Neath clouds of doubts and fears.
When desolation's chilling snows
   Would shroud the throbbing heart,
Amid the storm each blossom blows,
   And bids the clouds depart.

PERPETUAL BLOOM.

May He who hath ordained it thus,
   Still will it thus to be;
Till Life's uncertain streamlet glides
   Into Eternity!
And may Hope's blossoms, thus prepared,
   In realms beyond the tomb,
Freed from earth's blighting frosts and snows,
   Enjoy perpetual bloom!

HOLD ON!

Col. Crockett, renowned, very wisely hath said
    To his comrades in Life's valiant fight—
"Don't loiter along!—go ahead!—go ahead!
    But always be sure that you're right!"

And methinks that this motto so wise, might as well,
    By another cognomen be known;
Though cant, brief, and homely—wise counsel it gives—
    In the plain, simple language—" Hold on!"

Hold on to your heads when they'd nod their assent
    To what your hearts cannot approve;
Hold on to your tongues when they'd dare to defame
    The neighbor whom God bids you love!

Hold on to your principles—firmly hold on!
    When conscience declares that you're right,
Though legions of foes from within and without,
    Summon forth to a desperate fight.

Hold on to your feet when they'd lead you toward
   The grog-shop, or gambler's dark den;
Hold on!—and thus by an example so firm,
   Shield from error your weak fellow-men!

Hold on to your purse-strings when they would unclasp,
   To foolishly squander your store!
Hold on to your hands when such deeds they'd perform,
   As would bring you remorse, evermore!

Hold on to your hearts, young ladies, hold on!
   Don't love a moustache with such pains,
Till you feel quite assured the appendage has not
   Been donn'd to conceal lack of brains.

Hold on, also, young gents, hold on to your hearts!
   Till you're sure that the beauties you prize,
Are not only sustain'd in their freshness and youth (?)
   By the aid of Parisian dyes.

Ay! when error and sin and temptation assail,
   More than half of the conflict is won,
If our banner this motto unfurl to the gale—
   Be not over-hasty—Hold on!

THEY SLUMBER HERE.

THOUGHTS SUGGESTED DURING A VISIT TO THE BURIAL PLACE OF DEPARTED RELATIVES.

Tread lightly! This is sacred ground!
   The sainted dead are here!
Pass softly by each grassy mound
   That holds their relics dear.
Each little hillock robed in green,
   Awakes, within my heart,
The latent powers of memory,
   As with a magic art.

Why pause I here above this grave,
   With feelings sad and lone?
A mother's form lies buried here,
   Whose soul to God has flown;
While by her side, my honor'd sire
   In Death's embrace lies low,
No more to share the common lot
   Of mortals here below.

THEY SLUMBER HERE.

That grassy mound, apart from these,
    In silence lone, contains,
Reposing in a dreamless sleep,
    A grandsire's loved remains.
And one I loved in childhood's years,
    Rests here, beneath this sod;
In manhood's prime, his ransom'd soul
    Was summoned home to God.

While here, beneath this plain, white stone,
    There rests, in sweet repose,
The form of one who early left
    This scene of mortal woes;
She stood beside a manly form,
    A happy, trusting bride;
A twelvemonth lived to glad his home—
    Her first-born blessed—and died.

Fond mem'ry bids me linger now,
    Above another tomb,
And muse upon the lovely clay
    Reposing 'mid its gloom.
My sister-friend, so early called
    To slumber with thy God,
Permit me now to sadly muse
    Above thy covering sod.

Thou wast the last of this loved band,
    God summon'd to the skies;
Hence, fresher in my memory,
    Fond thoughts of thee arise,
I see thee as I saw thee, when,
    Upon that mournful day,
In speechless grief, we hung above
    Thy pale and lifeless clay.

I see thy glossy ebon hair
    Smoothed o'er thy marble brow,
Which, though the sun of life had set,
    Was beauteous, even now.
I see those death-dimmed orbs of thine,
    Once lit by love most true,
Veiled by those lids whose fringe caressed
    Thy cheeks of ashen hue.

And then I ask why one so fair,
    So lovely and beloved,
Should from these transient earthly scenes
    So early be removed?
It may be long ere I again,
    Unto these haunts may come;
For duty calls me far away,
    'Mid other scenes to roam.

THEY SLUMBER HERE.

But, wheresoever I may be,
 Whatever fate attend,
I'll muse upon the spot where rests
 Each fondly cherished friend.
And Heaven grant, that when this heart
 Hath ceased Life's busy strife,
I'll slumber in the arms of death,
 With those I loved in life.

HOME THOUGHTS.

CRYSTAL SPRING, PA.

Seated by the open casement,
   Fanned by pure and balmy air,
Gaze I on the distant landscape,
   Fraught with beauty, rich and rare;
Mark the clear and placid river
   Flowing onward toward the sea,
While the varied tints of Autumn
   Blend in lovely harmony.

And, anon, the locomotive,
   Bearing forth its pond'rous load,
Like a living thing of action,
   Thunders on the iron road.
While aloft, the magic wire,
   Gleaming in the sunshine bright,
Carries th' electric fluid,
   Morse's genius taught to write.

HOME THOUGHTS.

Now my restless musings wander
  To the days of long ago;
When yon river's sparkling wavelets
  Bore the Indian's canoe.
When the Indian maid her mirror
  Sought beside that crystal stream;
Or, beneath the forest shelter,
  Oft indulged in "Love's young dream."

And, though fervently my bosom
  Glows with patriotic pride,
At my country's growth and greatness,
  Now extending far and wide;
Yet, 'mid her primeval beauty
  Busy Fancy loves to roam,
With the noble-hearted red man,
  In his ancient forest-home.

Ere the unrelenting "pale-face"
  Had invaded his domains,
And he dwelt, in savage freedom,
  'Mid our valleys, hills, and plains,
Ere the poisonous "fire-water"
  To his wigwam had been brought,
By his "*more enlightened*" brother,
  Who his final ruin sought.

And, when musing o'er the changes
    Which Progression's hand hath traced,
In my mind the thought arises—
    Will these scenes e'er be effaced?
Will this present age of wonders,
    Judged by wiser heads than ours,
Vanish, 'neath the mighty conquest
    Of proud Genius' magic powers?

Vain the task to solve the problem—
    Future ages only can;
"Let us then be up and doing,"
    Working out Progression's plan!
But whatever be accomplished
    In the ages yet to come,
May Columbia e'er, and justly,
    Boast herself fair Freedom's home!

OUR SUNBEAM.

Ev'ry household hath its sunbeam!
   And, thank Heaven, we have ours;
Wooing, into life and beauty,
   'Mid earth's brambles, sweetest flowers.
Not a sunbeam from the golden
   Orb of day 'tis ours to share,
But a little cherub sunbeam,
   Shedding gladness everywhere.
Such a sunbeam as the Father,
   In His goodness, doth bestow;
Lest His children, overladen,
   Weary of life's conflict grow.

In and out, with ceaseless patter,
   Run the tiny little feet;
Tears and smiles of their possessor
   Alternating moments fleet.

Asking questions almost countless,
    With a pretty, arch resolve;
Questions that 'twould ofttimes puzzle
    A philosopher to solve.
Grateful are we for such sunbeams,
    Lighting this, our earthly way—
Heaven bless their future life-course—
    Heaven bless them all for aye.

OUR SHADOW.

Ev'ry household hath its shadow!
   And, alas! to ours have come
Shadows deep'ning, wid'ning, broad'ning,
   To the portals of the tomb!
Once a gem of rarest value
   In a fragile casket lay—
A pure spirit plum'd for Heaven,
   Scatt'ring o'er life's rugged way
Blossoms of such varied beauty,
   Pearls of such intrinsic worth,
That its Heaven-appointed mission,
   All too holy seemed for earth.

And the Spoiler came and scourged it,
   Marred its beauties, hour by hour;
Till that fair and fragile casket
   Prostrate lay beneath his power.
Then it was the shadow broadened
   Here beneath our homestead tree;

From a light, to us extinguished,
    Bright'ning in Eternity.
May that light, that angel pharos,
    Guide our storm-tossed barques to shore
Where the sunshine knows no shadow,
    Where the darkness comes no more.

THE ROOM WHERE LOVED ONES DIE.

We open it in sadness, and we close it with a sigh,
The door that guards the entrance of the room where
loved ones die.

The softly-sighing zephyrs float through that darkened room,
On pinions richly laden with delicate perfume;

The drowsy bees are humming around it all the day,
And feathered songsters warbling, as they flit from
spray to spray;

All nature seems inviting to scenes of festive joy,
To pleasures all unmingled with aught of an alloy;

Yet we open it in silence, and we close it with a sigh,
The door that guards the entrance of the room where
loved ones die.

There the last word was spoken; there the unsteady
    breath
Gave token of the presence of the ghastly king—
    stern Death.

The hand we clasped relaxing its slight and slighter
    hold,
First powerless grew, then pulseless, then stiff and
    icy cold;

The heart was stilled—the features grew placidly
    serene,
And the form we fondly cherished told but of what
    had been.

Such the associations that follow in their train,
As with melancholy pleasure we recount them o'er
    again;

As we open it in sadness, and close it with a sigh—
The door that guards the entrance of the room where
    loved ones die.

HEAVENLY TREASURES.

Treasures in the heavenly kingdom—
   A triumphant seraph band—
At the mandate of the Father,
   In His holy presence stand;
How they draw us! How they draw us!
   Treasures in that heavenly land.

How their subtle power magnetic
   Breaks the charms of earth away!
How their language, most prophetic,
   Tells us of our swift decay!
How they warn us! How they warn us!
   Bidding us to watch and pray.

Father, gathering in thy Kingdom
   Thus our treasures, one by one,
Some 'mid shadows of life's twilight,
   Others ere their transient sun
Reached its zenith, reached its zenith,
   Life's brief journey scarce begun,

Help us, wise and holy Father,
　　To regain those treasures there,
By a life of love and duty,
　　Faith, and hope, and earnest prayer!
Help us gain them! Help us gain them,
　　Where tried virtue knows no snare!

LET JEHOVAH JUDGE.

IMMORTAL toilers in life's harvest-field,
Binding the ripen'd grain its soil doth yield;
Ye who your soul's tribunal daily scan,
And seek the duty due from man to man;
Deal not too harshly with that stricken one
To whom hath set Hope's bright, alluring sun!
Gaze not too coldly on that care-worn brow!
Ye know not of the grief that lies below.

For, could ye trace the records of the Past,
The shadows dark which o'er that heart they've cast;
Could ye behold the penitential tears
In secret shed, 'mid hopes, and doubts, and fears;
Discern the causes for each trace of care,
That time-worn countenance doth sadly bear;
Ye could not coldly gaze upon that brow,
When ye beheld the grief that lies below.

LET JEHOVAH JUDGE.

Perchance some cherished friends, in Life's gay morn,
Were from that fond heart's tendrils rudely torn;
Perchance around it Love's deceitful chain
In some unguarded hour, was bound in vain;
Or from Religion's calm and placid ray,
Perchance the Tempter led it far astray;
Then gaze not coldly on that care-worn brow!
Ye know not of the grief that lies below.

For, thus may its most cherished joys have flown,
Before their fragile blossoms yet were blown;
Thus unrelenting Fortune may have frowned,
Shedding her blighting influence around;
Then leave to God that sad and stricken heart—
For He alone can sov'reign gracè impart—
And gaze not coldly on that care-worn brow!
Ye know not of the grief that lies below

CAST THY BREAD UPON THE WATERS.

"Cast thy bread upon the waters: for thou shalt find it after many days."—*Ecclesiasties* xi. 1.

"CAST thy bread upon the waters"—
  Pilgrim on life's thorny maze!
Cast it forth! and thou wilt find it—
  Find it after many days!
Look above, beneath, around thee!
  View the heavenly blessings strewn!
Teaching thee the noble lesson—
  Live not for thyself alone!

"Cast thy bread upon the waters,"
  Soldier on Life's battle-plain!
Cast it forth! in faith believing
  'Twill return to thee again!
He the boon of life deserves not,
  Who but for the present lives;
Failing to improve each moment
  God in His great goodness gives.

"Cast thy bread upon the waters!"
　　Freely it is given thee;—
Cast it forth! and thou wilt find it,
　　Find it in Eternity.
Though thou never mayst behold it
　　In thy pilgrimage on earth;
Heaven retains it to reward thee—
　　Faithful, fearless, cast it forth!

DYING EMBERS.

Have ye ever watched the embers,
   As they one by one depart—
Not upon a cheerful hearth-stone,
   But, within an aching heart?
Have ye marked the fitful flashes
   Darted forth ere life was o'er,
Till the dull and pallid ashes
   Told you that they lived no more?

Dying embers on a hearth-stone
   Is a cheerful sight to view;
But the heart's consuming embers
   Have for all a sombre hue.
Hearthstone fires may be replenished
   And rekindled in their turn;
For, unchanging laws in nature
   Bid them cheerily to burn.

But it was the heart's affections
　　Lighted first the embers there;
Only doomed to pale and glimmer
　　By repulsion's lurid glare.
All in vain they flash and lighten,
　　Liven'd by hope's cheering ray;
For, at last, that ray's extinguished;
　　And they slowly die away.

Weary mortals, in whose bosoms
　　Your heart's embers thus have died,
Be not fearful! Be not faithless!
　　Souls must thus be purified.
And, for you those ashen embers
　　Will rekindled be above;
Burning, with a flame undying,
　　In the realms of endless love.

LANDSCAPES OF LIFE.

WRITTEN ON NEW YEAR'S EVE, 1859.

To-night the Old Year dieth!
All day the restless earth, rob'd in the snowy shroud
That winter gives, has silently received
The crystal tear-drops Nature seems to shed
O'er his departure. Even now, methinks,
His fun'ral knell is rung by angel bands,
Who mark the flowing of the tide of time.
And, when the last faint echo dies away
Upon the midnight air, th' merry birthday bells
Will ring a welcome to the new-born year.

Wrapp'd in the visions of the buried past,
Almost unconscious of surrounding scenes,
My spirit's eye hath roam'd far, far away
Into the lapse of by-gone years. While mem'ry
With magic touch, portrays, in colors bright,
Landscapes of life, whose outlines faint, old Time
Has traced.

'Tis but a panoramic view
She gives; but oh, what 'membrance of past joys,
What shades of grief, they to my vision bring!
   First, 'mid those pictures bright, methinks I see
A cherish'd form my infant lips address'd
By the fond name of mother. Th' purest joys
My heart have ever thrill'd, were felt when
In th' sunshine of her smile; while the warm kiss
Imprinted on my cheek spoke love unfeign'd.
Such love, methinks, I never more may know,
Until this throbbing breast hath pulseless grown.
For, 'mid that 'raptur'd bliss the reaper—Death—
Bore her away among the priceless sheaves
The Father had declar'd fit for His garner.
They told me she had gone from earth for aye;
And though to childhood's view it seem'd a dream,
Its stern realities I since have felt—
An aching void within my heart, no form
But hers can fill, 'tis mine to know e'en now.
   That landscape bright, with all its leafy groves,
Its fragrant flowers and tesselated green,
Now fades away; and then another greets
My mental view. In this I recognize,
Beside my honor'd sire, the form of one
Who, I was told, had come to take the place

My bright "earth-star" had left. They told me
I must call *her* mother, too. I loved her well;
For she was good and kind. But yet, methought,
The love she bore to me was not so pure,
So deep, so fraught with nature's promptings,
As that of her who unto God had gone.
 I gaze upon the scene! and, as I gaze,
The sable hearse, the coffin, and the shroud,
Arise before me. While he, the guardian
Of my infant years, in manhood's prime,
Bows low beneath the icy touch of death,
And hastes to join his sainted partner
In the realms of bliss. 'Mid all these scenes,
In buoyancy of youth, fair, childish forms
Before me flit. Most prominent 'mong these,
Is one, a dark-eyed child, with ebon hair,
And her fair, blue-eyed sister. Hand in hand
We roam'd o'er hill and vale to cull spring-flowers;
In long, bright summer days we gleeful play'd
Beside the babbling brook; or sported with
The snowy robes of earth when winter ruled
The year. The hours of girlhood came; but yet
With hands unclasped, we trod life's path-way.

Our dark-eyed one before the altar stood—
I stood beside her there; saw the small hand
Resting confidingly in that of him
Her woman's heart had chosen. I heard
Those coral lips the promise breathe—to love
Till death should sever; and as she turn'd away,
Bright flowers seem'd strewn about her joyous path.
Rich blessings from the Father's hand were hers;
Yet, while the tendrils of our loving hearts
Clasped still more closely round that fragile form,
The yawning tomb received her lifeless clay. .
   Appalled we stood and gazed upon the wreck
Death's hand had wrought; and then, with aching hearts
And tearful eyes turn'd unto Him who gave,
And said : "Thy will be done!"
                          And thus, e'er since
Upon life's stream my fragile barque was launched,
Have those I lov'd the best been borne away
By some resistless current. Yet hath my course
Been fraught with blessings rife. True friends are mine—
Friends, *worthy of the name,* cheering me onward
Toward th' eternal port. And though life's landscapes

Might have been more bright—though in this brief
    review
Arise regrets for duties unperformed,
For moments unimproved; I thank my God
That His protecting care thus far hath kept
My wayward, wand'ring feet from error's path,
And made me what I am. I thank Him
For the blessings that are mine; and pray
That He may be my gracious Pilot still,
'Mid all life's storms. And when, at last, my barque,
Become too frail to longer cope with breakers,
Lies wrecked amid the shoals, may His
Redeeming love in safety guide
Its clay-freed tenant to the port of peace!

HOW SHALL WE KNOW THEM THERE?

"It doth not yet appear what we shall be: but we know that, when he shall appear, we shall be like him; for we shall see him as he is."—1 *John* iii. 2.

———

When these changing earth-scenes vanish from before the glazing eye,
When these fragile forms shall languish and with the cold earth-worm lie,
When the never-dying spirit seeks the mansions of the blest,
Freed from earth-stains to inherit God's eternal, promised rest,
When the loved ones, called before us, greet us in those mansions fair
With glad strains of sweetest welcome, how shall we discern them there?

HOW SHALL WE KNOW THEM THERE? 77

Will it be the form, the feature? Will it be the
    speaking eye?
Such endowments of the creature all too early fade
    and die!
Only to the soul immortal when life's silver cord is
    riven,
Entrance to those blissful portals was the sacred
    promise given.
Sown in nature and in weakness, raised in spiritual
    power,
Flesh and blood may not inherit ecstacies of that
    bright hour.

Says the evangelic writer—It hath not as yet been
    shown
What we shall be when we enter those blest realms
    to us unknown;
But we know when He appeareth to our sight no
    longer dim,
Clothed in His majestic beauty, we shall be like unto
    Him.
Sacred privilege, to be like Him—Him so spotless
    and so pure;
Who for human woes and frailties keenest suff'ring
    did endure.

Happy they who their affections base on spiritual worth,
Who, when the death-angel grants us freedom from the dross of earth,
And shall come that soul re-union pledged in the eternal sphere,
Shall not miss one grace nor beauty we have loved and cherished here!
Happy they! For moth, corruption ne'er their treasures can destroy—
Grant us Lord of earth and Heaven such a source of hope and joy.

'TIS HOME WHERE THE HEART IS.

" 'Tis home where the heart is!"—thus saith the poem—
" 'Tis home where the heart is, wherever we roam!
'Mid scenes of confusion, 'mid pleasure or pain,
In Sorrow's dark labyrinth—Fashion's gay train—
Whatever fond wishes our bosoms enfold—
If our search be for honor, for fame, or for gold—
Through whatever changes in life we may roam,
Wherever our hearts are—there—there is our home!"

Ask the fair child, as, in innocent glee
He roams through the forest glades, careless and free,
Or, sports in his gladness 'neath Heaven's high dome,
This soul-stirring inquiry!—Where is thy home?

He will point in reply to some pleasant retreat,
Where the friends of his childhood in harmony
    meet;
While, forth from his ruby lips, sweetly doth come
The words—" Where my mother is—there is my
    home !"

Ask the young wife as she stands by the side
Of him she has chosen her frail barque to guide;
To whom she has breathed the fond accents of love,
Which, though spoken on earth, are recorded above;
With a sweet, trusting smile she will quickly
    reply,
While a glance of sincerity beams from her eye
" Through whatever scenes my loved husband may
    roam,
Whatever his lot may be, that is my home !"

Ask the fond mother whose kindness and love
Are training her offspring for regions above !
Ask *her* her home, her heart's empire to show !
She will answer—" Wherever those loved ones may
    go;
In whatever station their lots may be cast,
In my hopes for the future, my joys for the past;

'TIS HOME WHERE THE HEART IS.

Amid whatever scenes those loved beings may roam,
With them will my heart be—with them is my home!"

Go ask the faithful instructor of youth,
As he guides, in the paths of fair science and truth,
Those beings, whose actions, for good or for ill,
Depend for success on his wisdom and skill!
In reply he will say—" 'Tis within Learning's halls,
Where the stern voice of duty impressively calls,
And points to where genius and talents have come,
Awaiting my counsel—there, there is my home!"

Go ask the seaman, who, o'er the blue sea,
Guides his proud vessel, swift, gallant, and free!
Say to him, when, safe on shore he has come—
Tell me, brave mariner! where is thy home?
In reply he will point you to old Ocean's wave,
Whose wild, stormy surges the sandy shores lave;
And say—" Where the billows cast high their white foam,
Where my ship rides in majesty, there is my home!"

'TIS HOME WHERE THE HEART IS.

Go ask the warrior, fearless and bold,
Who prizes Fame's laurels more highly than gold!
He'll direct you to where, on the wide battle-plain,
'Mid the groans of the dying his comrades are slain;
To where the wild war-trumpet sounds its alarms,
'Mid the roaring of cannon, the clashing of arms;
Where dangers are thickest, where dire perils come;
Within the broad battle-field—there is his home!

Go ask the Christian, who, 'mid toil and care,
Humbly the cross of his Saviour doth bear!
In true faith he'll reply—"In the regions of rest—
Those fair, happy regions, the realms of the blest—
Where bright-pinioned angels, where saints robed in white,
Sing praises unceasing by day and by night;
Where no sin, nor temptation, nor sorrow may come,
'Tis there that my heart is, yes, there is my home!"

Hath my poem a moral with sentiments true?
Or sketched in bright Fancy's bewildering hue?
Are we not daily taught by each station in life—
By the mother, the sister, the daughter, the wife,
By the warrior, seaman, or teacher so true,
That our hearts must be with us in all that we do?

Then, like the meek Christian whose home is above,
In the mansions of purity, goodness, and love;
'Mid whatever temptations or trials we roam,
In that land let our hearts be!—let that world be our home!

WITHOUT AN ENEMY.

Mortal, when life's scenes are ended,
    When its arduous toils are o'er,
When the 'franchised spirit gladly
    Anchors on the star-gemm'd shore;
Wouldst thou, while thy friends are mourning
    Over all earth claims of thee,
Have inscribed upon thy tomb-stone—
    Died without an enemy?

Oft we hear it, when the stricken
    Sorrow o'er the silent bier;
And perform the last sad duty
    Due to those they cherished here.
'Tis affection's voice that prompts it,
    And we would not harshly chide;
Though to claim such reputation
    Might not be our aim and pride.

WITHOUT AN ENEMY.

He who hath a *soul* within him,
　He who doth perform his part,
Ever faithful, ever fearless,
　In the world's exciting mart,
Must have enemies; the craven,
　Coward opposers of the right
Are the foes of *all* enlisting
　Boldly in Truth's earnest fight.

One who trod the purest life-path
　Ever trodden here on earth;
One who through a death triumphant
　Gave to man his second birth;
Even *He*, the God incarnate,
　Veil'd in mortal flesh to know
All the griefs of erring mortals,
　Had His enemies below.

For, say those who trace His records,
　" In the agonies of death,
Hanging with the malefactors,
　Ere He yielded up His breath;
By His friends denied, forsaken,
　By His enemies betray'd;
E'en amid these throes of anguish,
　For those enemies He pray'd."

Wouldst thou then, aspiring mortal,
    Die without an enemy?
Rather pray thy earthly life-course
    Like thy Master's may be free
From all error; ever striving
    Earnestly against the wrong;
And defending the defenceless,
    When they're injur'd by the strong.

Then, though enemies surround thee,
    Ever seeking to betray;
Trusting in the crown'd Redeemer,
    Falter not upon thy way!
But, like Him be ever praying,
    With a fervent heart and true—
Father, grant them Thy forgiveness!
    For they know not what they do!

THE FROST UPON THE PANE.

The golden sun has risen—all nature seems to wake,
And from night's gloomy prison her morning beams
    to take;
Our planet, clad in beauty, upon its course doth roll,
To waken thoughts of duty within the grateful
    soul;—
While o'er the fair creation steals Winter's icy train,
I gaze with admiration at the frost upon the pane.

Romantic scenes I'm weaving in that bright fairy-
    land,
And scarce the while believing they're wrought by
    Fancy's hand;
They tell of days departed, of joys no more to come,
When, gay and joyous-hearted, within my childhood's
    home,

I traced those figures airy and conn'd them o'er again,
And thought some graceful fairy had wrought them
    on the pane.

One morning, I remember, among the days gone-by,
One morn in cold December beneath a cloudless sky,
Awak'd from childhood's slumber, from out my
    trundle-bed,
I rose, and to my Maker my morning prayer said;
Then, turning to the window that brought day's
    beams again,
I there beheld with rapture the frost upon the pane.

In childish admiration my loving sire I sought,
And asked an explanation of what had there been
    wrought;
He fondly smiled upon me and strove, in accents
    kind,
To fashion proud philosophy to suit my infant mind;
I listened with intense delight—I could not long re-
    main
In ignorance of that fair sight—the frost upon the
    pane.

My soul with zealous ardor and interest did glow;
The truth—I could not doubt it! for *father said 'twas so:*
Still did my busy fancy paint images most fair,
With witching necromancy among the frost-work there;
For, e'en amid life's duties those scenes I trace again,
And revel in the beauties of the frost upon the pane.

REMINISCENCES.

Mother, I'm thinking of thee now,
    As when, in childhood's years,
Thy kind hand bath'd my youthful brow,
    And dried my childish tears. Dear friend,
        My transient, childish tears.

It seems a long, long while ago,
    Since that fond touch I felt;
Or since, to lisp my infant prayer,
    Morning and eve I knelt. Morning and eve
        To breathe my prayer, I knelt.

For, when too young to know thy worth,
    Death bore thee far away;
And left me on this weary earth,
    Without thy care to stray. Helpless and lone
        Without thy care to stray.

And mother, changes sad have come
  Upon my path since then;
And I have oft in secret yearned
  For thy loved smile again. Have yearned to see
    That kindly smile again.

They tell me of a sister's love,
  A brother's gentle power;
And whisper of fond friendship's ties
  To cheer each lonely hour. Ah, sacred ties,
    To cheer each lonely hour.

Yes, these are dear—I prize them all;
  But ne'er can I enshrine
Within my heart an image like
  That cherished one of thine. No image can
    Usurp the place of thine.

They say I'm cold—perchance 'tis true:—
  I would not dare deny;
For I have learn'd to check the love
  That in my heart doth lie. That love, dear one,
    Extends to thee on high!

And to the partner of thy cares—
  My father—loved so well—
Who soon was called to join thee, where
  The saints and angels dwell. That happy land,
      Where saints and angels dwell.

And oft, when sad and lonely here,
  I long for unfeigned love,
I fancy you, my parents dear,
  Look down from Heaven above. Look down
      And bless your offspring with your love.

Then I'll not mourn, if here below
  Your spirits guide my way;
And lead me through this vale of woe,
  To realms of endless day. Yes, safely guide
      To realms of endless day.

Enough to know that when on earth
  Life's silver cord is riven—
The orphan and the motherless
  Will be secure in Heaven. Blest and secure,
      With Jesus Christ in Heaven.

THE CHILD'S MATIN HYMN.

TRANSLATED FROM THE FRENCH OF LAMARTINE.

Oh, Father! whom my sire adores,
   To whom my mother humbly bows;
Whose name, breathed only on our knees,
   With terror and with sweetness glows.

'Tis said the bright and glowing sun
   Is but a plaything in Thy sight;
That underneath Thy feet 'tis hung,
   Like to a lamp of silver bright.

'Tis said Thou causeth to be born
   The birds within the fields so gay;
And giveth to the little child
   A soul to love Thee day by day.

'Tis said 'tis Thou who dost produce
   The flowers that in the garden grow;
And that without Thee—covetous,
   The orchard would no fruit bestow.

THE CHILD'S MATIN HYMN.

The bounties which Thy goodness gives,
    To all the Universe are free;
No insect is forgot, that lives,
    At this great banquet spread by Thee.

The lamb doth on the wild thyme graze,
    The goat the cytisus doth love;
To the urn's edge the little fly
    The white drops of my milk doth move.

The lark the bitter grain doth leave,
    And from the gleaner soars above;
The sparrow seeks the winnower—
    The child doth its kind mother love.

And, if the gifts Thou dost produce,
    We would each day from Thee obtain,
At morn, at evening and dawn,
    'Tis meet we should pronounce Thy name.

Oh, God! although my stamm'ring tongue
    Scarce speaks this name, by angels feared,
Within the holy choirs above,
    Even a little child is heard.

THE CHILD'S MATIN HYMN.

Oh, since from far He deigns to hear
    The vows that from our hearts proceed,
I'll ceaselessly demand of Him
    The heavenly gifts that others need.

My God, give waters to the fount—
    Give feathers to the sparrows small!
Give wool unto the little lamb—
    Cause dew upon the plains to fall!

Give health unto the suff'ring sick!
    Bestow upon the beggar bread!
Freedom unto the pris'ner give!
    Grant shelter to the orphan's head!

Upon the sire who fears the Lord,
    A numerous family bestow!
Grant grace and wisdom unto me,
    That peace my mother e'er may know.

GONE TO REST.

Gone to rest! these words, how soothing,
   Fall they on the mourner's ear;
As he bends, in speechless anguish,
   O'er the sad and solemn bier.

Death has come with his grim visage,
   And his sure unerring dart;
Stilled the quick pulse, chilled the life-blood,
   Hushed the lately throbbing heart.

Lowly lies the son and brother,
   Husband, father, neighbor, friend;
He has left earth for another
   World, where joys may never end.

While, beside his pale form, shrouded,
   Stand the dear ones, loved in life;
Gazing on that form beloved,
   That has ceased its mortal strife.

And, while musing on the virtues
  Which endeared him unto all,
Hope seems dying in each bosom,
  Sorrow doth each heart appall.

But a still, small voice, so cheering,
  Now pervades each throbbing breast;
Whispering, in gentle accents,
  He has sweetly gone to rest.

Stricken mourners, cease your sorrow!
  Hope and Faith do sweetly say—
" Wait ye for a brighter morrow!
  When, in realms of perfect day,

You may meet the dear departed,
  In the region of the blest;
'Mid the gentle and true-hearted,
  Who, with him, have gone to rest."

DESCRIPTION OF A WINTER MORNING.

A RIDE THROUGH HUNTINGDON VALLEY, MONTGOMERY COUNTY, PA. *Written by request,* ON NEW YEAR'S DAY, 1861.

'Twas morn—and o'er the vale of Huntingdon,
Shone forth, unclouded, the bright winter sun;
Dame Nature, having doffed her robes of green,
Clad in a spangled livery was seen;
Each object she presented, seemed to cheer,
And greet with radiant smiles th' infant Year.
O'er earth, a pure, unsullied sheet of snow
Concealed the Frost-king's ravages below;
While beauteous crystals in the sunlight shone,
Like glitt'ring icebergs in the polar zone;
Each evergreen whose beauty nought could blight,
Clothed in a spotless drapery of white;
Relieved by spangled robes of brightest green,
In soul-entrancing loveliness was seen;

DESCRIPTION OF A WINTER MORNING.

Each prancing steed that bounded swift along,
Neighing in concert with the sleigh bell's song,
Seem'd all-inspired with th' enliv'ning mirth
That ever cheers the denizens of earth;
When feath'ry snow-flakes from the clouds descend,
And, in one glitt'ring sheet of whiteness blend;
That morn one year ago, o'er Nature smiled,
And gladly welcomed her fair, infant child;
Who, calmly, yesternight, from earth-life free,
Launched on th' ocean of Eternity.
And now, another child to her is born,
Whose birth we hail on this auspicious morn;
A morn as bright, as full of wintry cheer,
As that which ushered in his brother year.
Thanks to kind Heaven for such scenes as these!
So fraught with beauty, and so formed to please;
For, gazing on these splendors, all unsought,
Which Nature's cunning artist here hath wrought;
Oh, who can say stern winter hath no charms,
When, folding closely in his frost-bound arms
Each rippling streamlet, shrub, and shady tree,
Now robb'd of their bright summer livery?
Each season hath its pleasures, beauties, too;
In turn unfolded to the ravish'd view;

And He who marks their changes as they roll,
This lesson teaches to the grateful soul—
From these, oh, man, from these unchanging laws
Learn to adore the great, primeval Cause;
And while His gifts His love unfolds to view,
Know that the bounteous Giver loves thee, too.

MY VOCATION.

Sitting in my quiet school-room,
    Fann'd by perfum'd summer breeze;
List'ning to the mirthful laughter
    Of the rompers 'neath yon trees;

I am now in soul transported
    'Mongst the merry, joyous train
Of youth's playmates; and seem living
    Happy school-days o'er again.

Now the school-bell loudly ringing,
    Calls each pupil to his seat;
Ceased the playing and the singing—
    Happy smiles my vision greet.

Slates and books and maps appearing,
    Now in turn each dear one cries—
"Tell me please what means this sentence,—
    Where these winding rivers rise."

MY VOCATION.

'Mid a host of varied duties,
    Thus each day and hour I move,
Sometimes irksome, always pleasant,
    In an atmosphere of love;

As each one his lesson conning,
    Claims assistance from my hand;
All the while obeying promptly,
    Cheerfully each just demand.

Fruit and flowers my desk adorning,
    Scent the balmy summer air;
Cull'd by childish hands each morning,
    Proffer'd me by young and fair.

Who will say the teacher's mission
    Is not one of hope and love?
Who will say no joys elysian
    Wait him in his home above?

Make me, oh, divinest Teacher,
    Faithful in my duties here!
Waiting my reward with patience,
    In a higher, purer sphere!

LUCK AND PLUCK.

*"What men call luck
Is the prerogative of valiant souls,
The fealty life pays its rightful kings."*—*J. R. Lowell.*

How much on this revolving sphere,
   That people term success,
Depends, not on the will of Fate,
   But the will which *we* possess;
And, though the world-wise connoisseur
   May boldly call it luck;
As boldly I the question ask—
   Friends, is it luck or pluck?

Your neighbor starts in business;
   He works and perseveres;
His gold and bank-notes fast increase
   With his increase of years;—
He basks secure 'neath fortune's smiles!
   The world exclaims—"What luck!"
But, is the world's decision right?
   Or, was it only pluck?

Another, by some sad mishap,
    His fortune all has lost;
For, far too hasty he has been,
    Nor paus'd to count the cost;
He tries again—seeks to avoid
    The rock on which he struck;
He soon becomes a millionaire—
    Say—was this luck, or pluck?

One, on the pathway to renown
    And honor, now would turn;
And nightly doth the midnight oil
    For him in secret burn;
He nears the pinnacle of fame!
    Earth's idlers deem it luck;
But, was it luck that placed him there?
    Or, an unyielding pluck?

Now, my opinion's briefly this:—
    No matter who agree;—
I make it known to one and all,
    Frankly and candidly,
That, though so much is often said
    Of good and evil luck,
What men call the decrees of Fate,
    Are rather pluck than luck.

I WOULDN'T BE JEALOUS, IF I WERE YOU.

Weary probationers, one and all,
Treading the face of this earthly ball,
Though your lot seems hard, and your irksome way
Grows rougher and darker every day;
If the ways of God you've not understood,
When the wicked have triumph'd above the good,
I'd scan such events with a closer view,
But I wouldn't be jealous, if I were you.

If your neighbor, by methods you can't explain,
Each day and hour seems wealth to gain;
And by means you do not understand,
Adds houses to houses, and land to land;
If his "loved ones at home" costly raiment have had,
While yours were in coarsest garments clad;
Don't let such events make your spirits "blue;"—
I wouldn't be jealous, if I were you.

106 I WOULDN'T BE JEALOUS, IF I WERE YOU.

If another more tact than you can boast,
Seeking his gain at another's cost;
And, by some most marvellous mystery,
To fame and honor seems rising high—
Seems gaining the acme for which you've wrought,
And with diligent efforts, yet vainly sought;
I'd honestly labor to gain it too—
But I wouldn't be jealous, if I were you.

If one with a beauteous form and face,
Endowed with every witching grace;
The observ'd of all admiring eyes,
Wins the devotion you so much prize;
If the flattering words that freely flow,
Should rouse in your bosom an envious glow,
I'd thank kind Heaven for blessings, too,
But I wouldn't be jealous, if I were you.

Ah, no! all these glittering toys of earth,
Eluding our grasp, are of little worth;
For did we but know the toil and pain
We must oft endure to secure such gain;
Methinks we would well-contented be
With what we have, and with what we see;
Then ever to God and yourself be true;—
But I wouldn't be jealous, if I were you.

CHILDHOOD'S HOME.

STANZAS SUPPOSED TO HAVE BEEN COMPOSED BY A LADY DURING A VISIT TO THE HOME OF HER CHILDHOOD, AFTER SEVERAL YEARS RESIDENCE IN THE WEST.—*Written by request.*

Beloved scenes of early youth,
    Once more you greet my gaze;
While mem'ry wafts me back again,
    To happy by-gone days;
To days when I, in childish sport,
    Roam'd o'er these fields so fair,
Protected by a mother's love,
    A father's guardian care.

And though, instead of lov'd ones, now,
    I stranger forms behold;
Familiar objects meet my gaze,
    Recalling days of old.

That quaint old house—the very same
  I cherish'd when a child;
The trees beneath whose shade I play'd,
  Fann'd by the breezes mild.

Yonder's the spring, the dear old spring,
  Whose waters oft I've quaff'd;
And ne'er will I again, I ween,
  Enjoy so sweet a draught,
As that which from its fountain flowed,
  When, in those joyous hours,
I wandered near its verdant banks,
  To gather woodland flowers.

The river winds as peacefully,
  As in those days of yore;
Its sparkling waves sport just as free
  Along its pebbly shore,
But, near its banks, its cherished banks,
  A change I now behold;
A scene that did not meet my gaze,
  Within those days of old.

Along the artificial road
  The burdened iron horse
Glides near the wires which testify,
  Of our immortal Morse.

CHILDHOOD'S HOME.

Why did I leave these rural haunts,
 In distant paths to roam?—
Forever dear thou'lt be to me,
 My loved, my childhood's home.

And when in the far West I join
 The friends who wait me there,
I'll picture oft these peaceful shades
 'Mid Nature's beauties rare.
Though it may never be my lot
 To visit them again,
Within my heart one treasur'd spot
 They ever will retain.

BIRTH-DAY PENCILLINGS.

Another link in his pond'rous chain
　Old Time has wrought for me;
And borne me, on his restless wings,
　Nearer Eternity.

Another page in life's mystic book,
　It now is mine to scan;
Then let me first each page review,
　Since I its cousre began.

And while I muse on that lifeless Past,
　Which its dead will not inter,
What a host of mem'ries, bright and sad,
　Within my bosom stir.

Forgiveness I'd extend to all
　Who've wronged me here below,
And ask that on them, blessings true
　Kind Heaven may bestow.

And when they act from motives pure
   As pearls on Truth's diadem,
May they ne'er be judged, as harshly judged,
   As mine have been by them.

For you, congenial spirits dear,
   Who, with a gentle hand,
Have sought my pilgrimage to cheer,
   Toward th' celestial land;—

For you I ask that choicest gifts,
   Shower'd by a hand divine,
May crown your earthly path with bliss
   Such as you shed o'er mine.

While, for myself, I would no more
   Of life's alloy secure,
Than He who formed this throbbing heart,
   Knows that it can endure.

I ask no high position here
   In the "militant church" below,
But, in the "triumphant church" above,
   Eternal bliss would know.

Then bear me safely, father Time,
    Upon thy restless wings;
Till Death shall bid my spirit soar
    From earth and earthly things.

And whether th' links that yet remain,
    For me be many or few,
May they more closely bind my soul
    To th' cross of th' Tried and True.

SUMMER CLOUDS.

Bright and beauteous summer clouds,
  Floating in the vault above;
Seeming like pure angel shrouds
  From the realms of light and love;—
Whence in beauty come ye now,
  Emblems of a brighter sphere;—
Flit o'er Heaven's azure brow,
  Then in silence disappear?

Are ye messengers of joy,
  From the regions of the blest;
Luring us from sin's alloy,
  Unto an eternal rest?
Proud Philosophy hath taught
  Both your mission and your cause;—
Trophies unto science brought,
  Governed by unerring laws.

But my wayward fancy oft
    Paints for you a higher source,
As I mark you float aloft,
    Gently on your destined course.
Heralds bright you seem to me,
    Chasing every shade of gloom,
Brightening each mystery
    Of the world beyond the tomb.

I remember, when a child,
    How I marked you gently part;
While imagination wild
    Revelled in my throbbing heart,
And, as you revealed to me
    Op'nings of an azure hue,
Eagerly I've watched to see
    Angel faces peeping through.

Now, when riper years have come,
    Chasing childhood's airy dream,
Emblems of a brighter home
    To my spirit still you seem.
Summer clouds, in beauty bright,
    Ever float aloft as now;
And, on airy pinions light,
    Flit o'er Heaven's azure brow!

TO MY NIECE ON HER NINTH BIRTH-DAY.

Thou cherished blossom, sent to bloom
   In Nature's garden fair,
Object of my unchanging love,
   And solace of my care;
My unassuming pen essays
   To trace these lines for thee,
Whilst I am musing o'er the Past—
   The Future's mystery.

Nine summers now have kissed thy brow—
   That brow so young and fair;
And yet, thy heart hath scarcely known
   A shade of grief or care.
A doting father's only pride—
   A mother's only joy,
Thy little barque doth smoothly glide—
   No breakers e'er annoy

But yet, light-hearted little one,
    Though now thy lot is blest,
We know not what dark shades of gloom
    May on thy future rest.
Nor need we know—I only ask
    Whate'er thy lot may be,
That strength sufficient for thy day
    Be granted unto thee.

I ask not wealth his costly gifts
    To lavish 'round thy home;
I ask not that thou mayst shine
    In Fashion's gilded dome;
I ask not Beauty fair to be
    Thy portion here on earth;
To tempt the sychophant to 'lure
    Thee from the homestead hearth.

But I would ask that wisdom pure,
    And virtue be thy lot—
That, 'mid each varied scene of life,
    Thy God be unforgot;
I ask that virtue, truth, and grace,
    May reign within thy heart;
And that thou mayst, in future years,
    Act the *true woman's* part.

TO MY NIECE ON HER NINTH BIRTH-DAY.

A few more days, and then, as wont,
  Thy form I may entwine,
And gently weave my hand among
  Those chestnut-curls of thine—
Till then, adieu! and when, on earth,
  Thy mortal course is run,
May angel hosts triumphantly
  Proclaim thy vict'ry won.

"GILPIN'S ROCKS."

CECIL COUNTY, MARYLAND.

ROMANTIC spot in Cecil's rural shade!
   My muse would fain pour forth her lays to thee;
For, 'mid thy rustic haunts I see portrayed
   The noble impress of the Deity:
'Twas on a sultry summer morn I sought
   Thy rugged rocks and brightly plashing spray,
With friends beloved, whose social converse, fraught
   With wit and wisdom, whiled the hours away.

Why did I sigh to linger 'mid thy scenes,
   When fleeting time bade me no longer stay?
Was it because bright Sol, with scorching beams,
   Shone forth effulgent o'er our destined way?
Was it because in leaving thee, I left
   Fond friends endeared to me by kindred ties;
Of their sweet converse soon to be bereft,
   While long and weary miles between us rise?

Yes, this in part!—But had I sought thy shades
   With no companion for my solitude,
I could have lingered long within each glade,
   And viewed each scene, majestic, wild, and rude.
Rock piled on rock in rural grandeur rise,
   While o'er them, bright and free, the waters play,
Shaded by trees, which, towering toward the skies,
   Obstruct th' entrance of each solar ray.

What work of art more beautiful and grand,
   Though wrought with finest touch of human skill,
Than this rude structure of th' Almighty's hand,
   Who fashioned it and formed it at His will?
To me, those wild and unfrequented scenes,
   The bounteous hand of Nature there displays,
Are far more beauteous than the painter's dreams,
   Revealed on canvass to th' admiring gaze.

Sweet spot, adieu! and though I never more
   May roam amid thy rustic haunts so fair,
Fond Memory must forsake her throne before
   I can forget thy beauties wild and fair.
For, like the friends who with me sought thy shades,
   Thy image is impressed upon my heart,
Never to be effaced by time or change,
   The freaks of fortune, or the works of art.

AUTUMN LEAVES.

Here, within my silent chamber,
   List I to th' Autumn rain,
As it falls with ceaseless patter,
   Gently on my window-pane;
While I gaze with admiration
   As th' earth the mist receives,
O'er the fair face of creation,
   At the bright-tinged Autumn leaves.

Autumn leaves—how wise a lesson
   Does their silent language teach—
With what eloquence impressive
   They to erring mortals preach!
Telling us that this world's pleasures,
   Fleeting, transient, are as they;
Warning us to place our treasures
   In the realms of perfect day.

AUTUMN LEAVES.

Autumn leaves, your dazzling beauty
  Calms the weary, troubled soul;
Leading it through paths of duty,
  To its God-appointed goal.
Harbinger of stern old winter,
  Soon you'll leave your parent bough;
Where ye cling in graceful clusters,
  Winning admiration now.

Meet it seems, that when the spirit
  Leaves its tenement of clay,
And is summoned to inherit
  Joys that will not fade away;
When our mother Earth's fair bosom
  Gently each pale form receives,
It should be when ye are fading,
  Bright and beauteous Autumn leaves.

THE SPIRIT-LAND.

> " Heaven is not far from those who see
> With the true spirit sight;
> But near, and in the very heart
> Of those who think aright."

WHY speak in such mysterious tones
　Of the far-off, spirit-land;
Where sing, in strains of music sweet,
　A happy, angel band?
Why gaze upon the azure sky,
　Smiling in beauty 'round;
And say—" Beyond yon ether fair,
　The Spirit-land is found?"

It may be that my thoughts are wild,
　And that they sometimes stray,
Like to a careless, wayward child,
　From their proper sphere away;

But oft methinks the Spirit-land
   Pervades the soul within,
When, deep within that soul, there lies
   No consciousness of sin.

When a Saviour's love doth reign supreme,
   Our errors all forgiven;
And His cheering smile in our spirits beam,
   This, this, I say, is heaven.
I would not doubt that Holy Writ
   Which describes those realms so fair;—
The crystal fountains, the golden gates,
   And th' bright-winged seraphs there.

But yet methinks if we ever would
   That blissful world attain,
Those happy scenes must be felt within,
   Ere its portals we may gain.
Far, far above us may be that sphere,
   Where our spirits freed may roam;
Yet these souls from sin must be ransomed here
   To enjoy so bright a home.

GOD MADE US TO BE HAPPY.

Canst thou doubt it? Look around thee
   See each fruitful, verdant field,
Telling of the bounteous harvest
   It will to the tiller yield.

Look upon the crystal waters!
   Listen to each songster's note!
As he warbles forth his praises
   Sweetly from his tuneful throat!

See all animated nature
   Sporting in the sun's bright rays;
Giving to their wise Creator
   Humble thanks and grateful praise!

View the azure vault above thee,
   Spangled with each sparkling gem!
Far more brilliant, far more lovely
   Than the monarch's diadem.

GOD MADE US TO BE HAPPY.

View these scenes, thou child of sorrow,
  And from them a lesson learn!
Yet on thee a brighter morrow
  Fortune's varying hand may turn.

Put thy trust in Him who made thee—
  Placed thee in this beauteous world!
Let no trials e'er dismay thee!
  Keep hope's banner wide unfurled!

He designs His erring children
  To be happy here below;
Though he sometimes dregs our gladness
  With the bitter drops of woe.

Yet, remember, fellow-traveller
  To the same appointed goal,
That he gives us these afflictions
  But to purify the soul!

Onward in the path of duty
  Let thy footsteps firmly press!
And thou early wilt discover,
  'Tis the road to happiness.

FUGITIVE LAYS.

FOR OAK LAWN, MONTGOMERY COUNTY, PA.

I'm thinking of a winsome spot
    Full many miles away;
Around which bloom, in sweet perfume,
    Bright flowers and blossoms gay.
In Autumn, in luxuriant pride,
    Among their leaves of green,
Are purple grape and velvet peach
    In rich profusion seen.

In winter, when the crested snow
    Whitens each hill and vale,
The cheering blaze within doth bid
    The haughty frost-king quail.
I'm thinking, too, of loved ones there,
    As busy mem'ry roams;—
Of those whose smiling faces cheer
    One of my earthly homes.

For I have many homes below,
    If (as the poet says)
Our home is found wherever glow
    The true heart's brightest rays,
Where warmest welcome waits us, when
    We to its threshold come;
If this be true, 'tis mine to claim
    Many an earthly home.

And this is one—this winsome spot
    Full many miles away—
For it the bright Forget-me-not
    Blooms in my heart for aye.
Upon this pleasant summer eve
    My fancy wanders there;—
Ye sighing zephyrs, on your wings
    My kindest wishes bear.

Oh, bear them to the cherished friends
    Who cluster 'round that hearth;
Whose sympathizing kindness cheers
    My pilgrimage on earth.
And may their future lot be blest
    As they have blest mine own!
May theirs be an eternal rest,
    'Mid joys earth hath not known!

Beloved friends, your 'membrance dear
　　Illumes life's rugged way;
God bless you in your sojourn here!
　　God bless you all for aye!
But ah! the waning hours forbid
　　This converse sweet with you;
For sterner duties wait me now;—
　　Ye gentle ones, adieu!

CURLING SMOKE.

O'er a landscape bare and brown,
   Blasted by the frost-king's stroke;
Rising from the busy town,
   See the graceful, curling smoke!

Yesternight the atmosphere
   Bade it sink unto the earth;
Now it soars through ether clear,
   Toward the realms of higher worth.

Upward, from consuming flames
   Takes it its etherial way;
Purpled by the golden rays
   Of the setting "king of day."

Like a thing of witching grace,
   On its heav'nward course it goes;
How I love that course to trace,
   'Mid these seasons of repose!

Spirit whom the saints invoke,
  Unto whom we bow the knee,
Upward, like the curling smoke,
  Henceforth let my life-course be.

FIDELITY.

*"False to the living, if thou wilt,
But faithful to the dead."*

FALSE, didst thou say?—Oh, no!—All nature speaks
And bids thee to recall those random words;
Lest in some trusting heart they cause a wound
No earthly balm can heal.
        Order, the great, first, truest law of Heaven,
Controlling all things in the Universe,
In silent language hourly doth proclaim
Its Legislator true, immutable.
And should not all that emanate
From that unchanging source, be as unchang'd—
As faithful to their trust as He whose word
Gave them existence here?
        True, human nature,
Unlike the Divine, more prone to error is;
More wont to stray from the appointed course.

Yet, He who formed that nature knows, full well,
How, in His own appointed time and way,
It may accomplish its life-given design.
        Oh, let us then be faithful unto all!
Yet, if we must be false, let it not be
Unto the living—those whose throbbing hearts,
Keenly alive to ev'ry painful wound
The poison'd arrows of neglect produce,
Shrink from their aim, as does th' sensitive plant
From the rude touch of mortals! No! rather let
The unconscious dead be victims unto
Our inconstancy. Yet they a claim possess—
A sacred claim on our fidelity.
And, from their earthy graves, their silent
Tongues, bound in death's icy fetters, seem
To speak, and hourly bid us to be false
To none.
        Then strive, oh, mortal man,
In all thy actions with thy fellows here,
One virtue more to add unto the list
By Holy Writ prescribed; and let that
Virtue be—*Fidelity*.

COME UP HIGHER.

Bright Sol's last rays had kissed the earth,
  The twilight hours drew near;
And gentle Luna's pearly rays
  Illumed our nether sphere.
The flowers had closed their petals fair,
  Gemm'd by the dew-drops bright;
While ling'ring day-beams yielded to
  The sombre shades of night.
The stars in beauty shone above;
  All nature did conspire
To fill the grateful soul with love
  And bid it come up higher.

Beside a couch a mother sat,
  In agony of grief;
No lovely scene without could give
  Her burden'd heart relief.

For near her lay a suff'ring child,
    Her only joy and pride,
Sinking beneath the stormy waves
    Of Jordan's swelling tide.
"Mamma," it said, "I dreamed, just now,
    Of God's seraphic choir;
They spread their snowy, glitt'ring wings,
    And bade me come up higher!"

The voice is hushed; the quick pulse stilled;
    The life-blood ceased to flow;
The fring'd lids are closed for aye
    On objects here below.
Death's damps are 'mid those clust'ring curls;
    That cherub form is still;
Those rounded limbs no longer move
    At childhood's earnest will.
A form lies there in Death's embrace,
    That angels might admire;
A soul has yielded to the call—
    "Pure spirit, come up higher!"

"Daughter," a skeptic father said,
    "Cast that dull book aside!
Believe me it was ne'er designed
    Our path through life to guide."

COME UP HIGHER.

"Papa, I cannot it renounce,
   While an immortal soul
Thus struggles 'mid its foes to reach
   Its God-appointed goal.
I love the holy prophet's zeal
   Waked by the Psalmist's lyre;
They call forth all that's pure and good,
   And bid me come up higher!"

"How know you an immortal soul
   Thus struggles with its foes;
And longs to reach a destined goal
   Exempt from earthly woes?"
"A something tells me it, papa,
   I feel it glow within,
It fain would burst its prison bars,
   And flee this world of sin.
In dark temptation's hour it glows,
   With ardent, pure desire;
It loathes its tenement of clay,
   And longs to soar up higher."

A youth, upon whose brow was stamped
   Th' impress of a soul
Awake to noble acts and deeds,
   Once sought the pois'nous bowl.

For Fortune with a threat'ning frown
   His path in life beset;
While dire Temptation lured him on
   To drink—"drink and forget!"
He sought the bowl, but turned aside;
   He quench'd the mad desire;
For conscience' "still, small voice," he heard—
   It whispered—"Come up higher!"

Thus, when temptation's syren voice
   Would 'lure the soul astray,
And bid us seek true happiness
   In sin's dark, thorny way;
When sorrow's cup 'tis ours to drain,
   When friends and fortune flee;
When th' o'erburdened, care-worn heart,
   Sinks in despondency;
Faith points to th' unnumber'd host
   Of Heaven's angel choir;
While hope smiles in the fainting soul,
   And bids it "come up higher!"

Comrades in truth's celestial cause,
   Let this our motto be!
Let us press onward to attain
   Our highest destiny!

COME UP HIGHER.

Justice and Right now lead us on,
    While Duty points the way,
Through sunlight dimm'd by ebon clouds,
    Unto a brighter day.
Life, health, and vigor now are ours,
    While all around conspire
To urge us on to victory,
    And bid us come up higher.

Then let no grov'ling thoughts be ours!
    Let virtue be our aim!
Let all that's noble, just, and true,
    Our fixed attention claim!
Where Duty calls, press bravely on!
    Nor ever disobey!
But, with determined, earnest zeal,
    Pursue our destined way.
And, when Death frees the fettered soul,
    May the angelic choir
Smile sweetly on us from above,
    And whisper—"Come up higher!"

RIPPLES IN THE GRAIN.

The summer sun, declining, his beams is darting free;
In gorgeous splendor shining o'er woodland, stream, and lea;
A moment still, he lingers at the portals of th' West,
And then, with rosy fingers, folds its drap'ry o'er his breast;
His luster, still adorning the clouds which hover there,
Casts rays like early morning, athwart a landscape fair;
And, as he sinks to slumber, the ev'ning zephyr train
Awakes, in countless number, the ripples in the grain.

RIPPLES IN THE GRAIN. 139

A sight of grace and beauty those ripples are to r
Portraying life's great duty on thought's tumultu
    sea;
They tell of pure emotions within the human breast,
When th' hour of calm devotion hath still'd the soul's
    unrest;
Foretell, in language truthful, the joyous harvest-
    time,
When sturdy yeomen youthful, with song, and jest,
    and rhyme,
Come forth in gleeful numbers, a merry reaper
    train,
T' break th' restless slumbers of th' ripples in the
    grain.

Great Father, 'mid thy blessings, oh, teach us all to
    know
The all-important lesson—from whence those bles-
    sings flow;
From earth's enchanting beauties, oh, may we ev'ry
    day,
Learn something of earth's duties upon our destined
    way;
And, as each harvest greets us, may it the truth
    renew—

That Thy great harvest waits us, and laborers are
 few !
While, flits each pure emotion in an angelic train,
Through thought's tumultuous ocean, like ripples in
 the grain.

GONE BEFORE.

*"Part of the host have crossed the flood,
And part are crossing now."*

Yes, part have crossed the flood, and safely stand
  Triumphant on the starry shore of heaven;
Within the confines of that blissful land,
  From Pisgah's top to Moses' vision given.

Methinks I see them now—the young, the gay—
  Manhood, with buoyant tread, and woman's form;
And aged veterans, whose locks of gray
  Wave in the winds of Death's portentous storm.

I see them as I saw them e'er they crossed
  The threat'ning waves of Jordan's swelling tide;
And mingled with that pure unnumber'd host,
  By th' inspired Evangelist descried.

Long years have passed since, by " the boatman pale,"
    Some of these voyagers were borne away;
While others, ere this Spring's reviving gale
    Had fanned their brows, left earthly scenes for aye.

One, frank, and free from all deceptive arts,
    And blithe and gay as lark from woodland flown,
Left us, when the fond tendrils of our hearts
    Were clasping close and closer to her own.

In vain a parent's, brother's, sister's, love
    Bade her remain and share terrestrial bliss;
Her spirit, lured to brighter worlds above,
    Burst from the bonds that fettered it to this.

Friends, sympathizing friends, with tearful eyes,
    Gazed on the scene, disheartened and appalled;
But, all unheeding, Jordan's waves arise—
    She could not linger when her Saviour called.

Another one, in early womanhood,
    'Mid all the cares of mother and of wife,
Whose soul bore impress of the true and good,
    Ent'ring Death's barque, forsook the shore of life.

An infant's wail, a prattling child's caress,
   The sobs of weeping friends assembled 'round,
A loving husband's look of tenderness—
   Nought, nought could stay that spirit " homeward bound."

These were the last on which my sorrowing eyes
   Gazed, as they neared the port of endless rest—
Mourning, yet joying that, in Paradise,
   " Th' early called are ever early blessed."

" And some are crossing now "—upon that stream,
   That cold, resistless, overwhelming tide,
'Mid winter's cold or summer sun's bright beam,
   The " boatman pale " his barque doth ever guide.

We near the margin, too. Thou Crucified,
   Oh! grant, that when for us that barque is steer'd;
We'll safely anchor on the other side,
   Though life-winds oft its destined course have veer'd!

May-day, 1860

CHARITY.

"You look very happy!" said Hilda to a penitent, who had just received the benediction of the priest. "Is it then so sweet to go to the confessional?"

"Oh, very sweet, my dear signorina!" answered the woman. "My heart is at rest, now. Thanks be to the Saviour, and the blessed Virgin, and the saints, and this good father, there is no more trouble for poor Theresa!" *Hawthorne's Marble Faun.*

PROTESTANT brother—thou who wouldst condemn
Each earnest action of thy fellow-men;
Simply because such actions, as thou saith,
Ignore what seems to thee a truer faith;
Oh, pause 'mid thy unjust severity,
And humbly learn a world-wide charity.

For, is not he who bows before his priest,
Feeling that of all saints he is the least,
Who through the Virgin would the Son revere,
Because unworthy to approach more near;

CHARITY.

Say—is not such as he closely allied
Unto the Publican Christ justified?

Then let us not our soul's Shechinah dim,
By thanking God that we are not like him;
But let us meekly forth our life-cross bear,
Nor lay it down until our crown we wear;
Nor, like to the self righteous Pharisee,
Vainly make broad our own phylactery.

And, when, in sin's dark vale thy brother strays,
Like a lost sheep, from virtue's pleasant ways,
Let not thy tongue, in cold, unfeeling scorn,
Add to the poignant grief already borne;
Remembering that the sinless shall alone
Presume to cast the contumelious stone.

For what to man is the "church militant,"
But that which soothes the lowly penitent,
Which bids all dogmas, creeds, and forms take flight
'Neath th' effulgence of the Gospel light;
Bears with our brother's frailties as our own,
And aids his progress towards the Father's throne?

The zealous Paul these duties all foresaw,
When seeking to expound this righteous law—
Now charity, faith, hope abide, said he;
But, greatest of them all, is charity;
And he who fails that charity to show,
Bliss in the "church triumphant," ne'er may know.

THE OLD HOMESTEAD.

There is a spot, a quiet spot, within a shady bower
Which holds within my heart, e'en now, a sway of
    magic power;
Far from the dusty highway's din, it stands in sweet
    repose;
A grassy by-way leads us where, long years ago, it
    rose:
And there, beneath the rural shade, so prized in days
    of yore,
An edifice of ancient art the stranger may explore,
It tells me of the friends beloved, who thronged those
    wide old halls,
And to my fancy once again each cherished scene
    recalls;—
'Twas there my sire my mother wooed; 'twas there
    he told his love;
'Twas there their mutual vows were pledged and reg-
    istered above;

And o'er that homestead's threshold dear, that gentle being passed,
To share the joys and cares of him with whom her lot was cast.
There too, in childish glee, I trod those antique oaken floors;
There, in the little yard I played beside those massive doors—
Familiar scenes, ye haunt me still; though weary years have flown,
And death hath sever'd me from friends I loved, and called my own.
My honored grandsire's hoary locks—methinks I see them now;—
That vigorous, athletic form, age sought in vain to bow;
Those kind and gentle tones of his, that firm, unyielding will;
Which, while he mildly chid my faults, proved that he loved me still;
The eight-day clock, so old and quaint, beside the chimney-piece,
Whose warning sounds so often bade my evening pastimes cease;

The orchard with its tempting fruits; the garden,
    richly stored;
The barn, designed from winter's storms the golden
    grain to hoard;
The spring-house and its dairy-maids, with faces
    bright and fair,
Its butter and delicious cream which 'twas my lot to
    share;
Those scenes I yet remember well, though many a
    change hath come,
And strangers now frequent the haunts where I was
    wont to roam.
Yes, cherished spot, this constant heart will hold
    thee still the same!—
Old places have a charm for me, the new can never
    claim;
And wheresoever I may be, whatever fate be mine,
I'll cling with fondness unto those endearing scenes
    of thine.
Christ teach me so to live, that when life's silver
    cord is riven,
I may enjoy with friends beloved, a homestead sweet
    in Heaven.

SUMMER FRIENDS.

"It was not an enemy that reproached me; then I could have borne it."—*Psalms* lv. 12.

Gazing from my western casement,
　　As the light with darkness blends,
Muse I on the Past and Present,
　　Muse I now on summer friends.

In the ether, clouds are lowering;
　　Darkly o'er my head they roll;
Thus are gloomy clouds of sadness
　　Lowering in my inmost soul.

Harshly blam'd have been my actions,
　　Earnest efforts to do good;
While my purest, best intentions,
　　Coldly have been misconstrued.

SUMMER FRIENDS.

Yet, methinks I might have borne it,
    Had it been mine enemy,
Who my life-path thus hath darkened
    With the shades of contumely.

But it was my guide, acquaintance,
    Whom I valued as a friend;
Whose good name and reputation
    Even now I would defend.

Why, then, do they judge thus harshly?
    Why expect me to confess
To internal thoughts and feelings
    I would shudder to possess?

I must doubt where once I trusted;
    Learn to shun where once I loved;
For that trust's unworthy objects
    False to friendship's pledge have proved.

Yet, 'tis best: I know, I feel it:
    E'en amid this deep'ning gloom
Brooding o'er my troubled spirit,
    Thus doth consolation come—

"While prosperity's bright sunlight
  Bade all praise and none to blame,
Thou beneath its influence basking,
  Scarce knew whence the blessing came.

"But these adverse gales, now blowing,
  Bring to view thy real friends;
And thou'lt value far more highly
  Those blest gifts the Father sends.

"And they'll draw thee closer, nearer,
  To thy faithful Friend above;
Bid thee place thy dearest treasures
  In the regions of his love."

Father, reigning in Thy kingdom,
  Though my erring fellow-men,
My sincerest, purest motives
  May unfeelingly condemn;

Thou who know'st my spirit's secrets,
  Who my thoughts can understand,
I would claim at Thy tribunal
  Truest justice at Thy hand.

Then, when life's alluring sunshine
 Ceases with its storms to blend,
May my soul, o'er death triumphant,
 Thank Thee for each summer friend!

"FAITHFUL IS HE THAT CALLETH YOU."

1 Thess. v. 24.

Little child, with careless glee,
Sporting on the flowery lea;
Maiden with the sunny hair,
Unto whom life seems so fair;
Youth with buoyant step and light,
Climbing fame's alluring height;
From earth's pleasures turn awhile!
Seek the path that leads from guile!
Seek the Holy and the True—
"Faithful is He that calleth you."

Matron, on whose brow serene,
Care's sad traces may be seen;
Manhood, 'mid whose locks of brown,
Threads of silver have been strewn,
Hoary age, whose bowing form
Soon will yield to life's rude storm;

From earth's trials turn away!
Seek Religion's inborn ray !
Seek the Holy and the True—
"Faithful is He that calleth you."

Soldiers of the sacred cross,
Ever counting all things loss,
For the knowledge ye have known,
Of the meek and lowly One ;
Toilers on life's battle-plain,
Where Truth's champions are slain,
Falter not when death shall come !
In Christ's kingdom there is room ;
Seek the Holy and the True !—
"Faithful is He that calleth you."

THE THREE SOLILOQUIES.

Heart, to me the truth unfold!—
   Heart, with anxious feelings fraught—
Am I dazzled by his gold?
   Do I love or do I not?

Is that brightly-flashing eye,
   Or that voice of winning art,
Graceful form or forehead high,
   Empire for a woman's heart?

Harry May they say is plain;
   Plain, alike in face and form;
Yet his bosom doth contain
   Pure affections, true and warm.

Truer far they seem to me,
   Than the haughty Darnley's love;
Yet, I've promised his to be,
   'Neath those stars that shine above.

THE THREE SOLILOQUIES.

God forgive me, if I sin,
    For my friends approve my choice;
Crush my fondest hopes within,
    Bid me 'mid my woes rejoice.

*   *   *   *   *   *   *

It is o'er—the word is said;—
    I am Horace Darnley's bride;—
My affections are betrayed—
    Fetter'd by a parent's pride.

Little thought that joyous crowd,
    Decked in costly jewels bright,
Who, with aspect coldly proud,
    Throng'd around me yesternight;

How that fragile bridal wreath
    Pressed upon my throbbing brow,
As I vow'd to love, till death,
    One I love not, even now.

How, as like a statue cold,
    I beheld the guests depart;
That each snowy satin fold
    Trembled o'er an aching heart.

But, 'tis done—the die is cast—
   I must try to love him now;—
Buried in the hidden Past
   Is each falsely utter'd vow.

*   *   *   *   *   *   *

Years have passed—three weary years,
   Since my childhood's home I left;—
Tears I've shed—aye, bitter tears,
   Of its peaceful joys bereft.

Costly equipage is mine;
   Servants wait in livery;
I, in silks and jewels shine,
   Doom'd to splendid misery.

Worldlings gaze with envious eyes,
   And esteem my station blest;
Fancy I have won a prize,
   In the wealth by me possess'd.

Would they had my paltry gold;—
   Would they had my princely home—
Father! from Thy peaceful fold
   Let thy lambkin cease to roam!

All my happiness while here,
   Sacrificed at mammon's shrine;
Own me in a brighter sphere!
   Bless me by Thy love divine!

"GOD TEMPERS THE WIND TO THE SHORN LAMB."

Stranger, whom Fate decrees to roam,
Far from thy native land and home;
Whose yearning soul ne'er sweetly blends
In social intercourse with friends;
When thy sad breast's internal pulse
Is quick'ning 'neath each rude repulse;
Approach the throne of the great I Am!
He "tempers the wind to the shorn lamb."

Mother, whose throbbing bosom yearns
For that wayward son who no more returns;
Who, 'mid ardent hopes and anxious fears,
Patiently watch'd o'er his infant years;
Who, with tearful eyes and aching heart,
Saw him from th' threshold of home depart;
Approach the throne of the great I Am!
He "tempers the wind to the shorn lamb."

GOD TEMPERS THE WIND TO THE SHORN LAMB.

Orphan, with tearful, downcast eye,
Whose soul is yearning for sympathy;
When th' heartless world with threat'ning frown
Doth weigh thy spirit with anguish down;
When thou art weary, sad, and lone,
Craving the love thou once hast known;—
Approach the throne of the great I Am!
He "tempers the wind to the shorn lamb."

Mourner o'er that departed worth,
Whose casket, within the silent earth,
Lies buried 'neath the valley's clod,
While its priceless jewel is flown to God!
Look through thy tears with an eye of faith!
Lo! ransomed saints to thy spirit saith—
"Approach the throne of the great I Am!
He 'tempers the wind to the shorn lamb'"

Ay, every weary, way-worn soul,
Trembling and faint ere you reach your goal,
Though winds may toss your frail life-barque,
And bear you afar from Safety's ark;
Still, as of old, your Saviour's nigh,
Whisp'ring softly—"Fear not, 'tis I!"
Approach the throne of the great I am!
He "tempers the wind to the shorn lamb."

UNDER-CURRENTS.

FONDLY INSCRIBED TO MY FRIEND, "KATHLEEN."

KATHLEEN, my friend, dost thou remember when
    Once we together rode through Buckingham?
Pass'd one by one the neat abodes of men,
    In rural ease reposing, still and calm?
A tempest was before us—not a storm:
    Ah, no! for wintry winds blew soft that day;—
But one of *Equus'* race, whose noble form
    Envelop'd in his coat of dapple-gray,
Safely toward Doylestown bore us on our way.

Incessantly we chatted; women do
    On all occasions—so, presuming, say
" Creation's lords;" and whether false or true,
    For once, at least, we'll let them have their way.
Now gay, now serious, conversation's tide
    Flow'd forth unchecked as moments glided on;
We spoke of friends in girlhood's, manhood's pride,

Whose brief heart histories we each had known,
And from whose bosoms much of life's best hopes
  had flown.

And then, in thy own, unassuming style,
  This language thou to me addressed, Kathleen :—
"I sometimes think that many, all the while
  Cold, unimpassion'd they to others seem,
Conceal an under-current in their breast,
  Known but to him who formed the human heart ;
A current causing oft that heart's unrest,
  As calmly, patiently they bear their part
In this world's unrelenting, cold, and selfish mart."

So true thy language seemed, it made vibrate
  Each hidden cord within my inmost soul ;
And many times I've thought—how pure, how great
  The joy of those must be, who reach life's goal
Free of such currents. Then again I pause ;
  Knowing that He, the author of our life,
Kindly directs by His unvarying laws
  These inner streams with restless waters rife,
To find their source in Him the one great Fount of
  life.

Proud Science in th' outer world doth give
    Reasons for under-currents of the sea;
But for the spirit's surgings we'd receive
    A more profound and pure philosophy.
For who can tell the deep, internal woe
    Of souls who bear these under-currents forth?
Who but th' omniscient One may ever know
    Their secret longings, 'mid the scenes of earth,
For something formed of more enduring worth?

Mayst thou, my friend, if thy young life has e'er
    Been fraught with deep emotions such as these;
The anchor place of thy aspirings, where
    No storm shall scathe it—where no gentler breeze
May sway its cable; and mayst thou e'er know—
    Acting thy part in earth's mysterious scene—
Hearts as impressible of others' woe,
    Friends true to thee as thou to thine hast been!
May Heaven bless thy lot, as now, for aye, Kathleen!

IMPROMPTU TO WATER.

Dame Nature fair
Hath beauties rare
  To charm each son and daughter;
But nought that she shows
With more beauty glows
  Than the pure and limpid water.
Like diamonds bright,
In the warm sunlight,
  It sparkles in stream and river;
In seeming glee
It gurgles free—
  This gift of the bounteous Giver.

In waves it rolls
Toward th' icy polls,
  'Mid the depths of the surging ocean;
Or, reckless falls
O'er some rugged walls,
  Rent by the earth's commotion.

It dances along,
To th' mermaid's song
　　Of joy, joy now and ever;
Ne'er its beauty dies
'Neath th' wintry skies;
　　For its charms it retains forever.

The flowers meet death,
When th' blighting breath
　　Of the frost-king breathes upon them;
And the trees and grass,
As they mark him pass,
　　Seek their sombre robes to don them.
But the water, though
It may cease to flow,
　　In its laughing summer beauty,
Hath never yet
Seem'd to quite forget
　　That its is a joyous duty.

In snowy flakes
From the clouds it breaks,
　　When icy chains have bound it;
And gracefully falls
From its lofty halls
　　To enliven the gloom around it.

Then, in stainless drifts,
Its form it lifts
  As the sleigh-bells merry tingle,
With loaded sleighs
And charger's neighs,
  Pass by with varied jingle.

When each stream, frost-bound,
Shows to all around
  The skill of the wise Creator,
Their surfaces yield
An ample field
  For the feet of the joyful skater.
Thus the water bright,
Like a fairy sprite
  In its varied forms of beauty,
Hath never yet
Seem'd to quite forget
  That its is a joyous duty.

I value them all,
Both great and small—
  These gifts of the bounteous Giver;
Yet, for me, I confess,
None such charms possess
  As this spirit of sea and river.

IMPROMPTU TO WATER.

Ay, Nature fair
Hath beauties rare
   To charm each son and daughter;
But nought she shows
With more beauty glows,
   Than the pure and limpid water.

TO THE SCHUYLKILL RIVER.

Sweet Schuylkill, my own native stream,
    To thee my strains belong;
Be thou my humble muse's theme—
    The subject of my song.

Though bards have seldom sung of thee
    In measure or in rhyme;
Thou'lt hold, within my memory,
    A place throughout all time.

Thou canst not boast fair Hudson's scenes,
    Nor Delaware's broad waves;
Nor wouldst thou admiration win
    Where Susquehanna laves.

But, though beside thy sister streams,
    Thou humble dost appear;
Thy name will ever be to me
    Most sacred and most dear.

For, 'twas upon thy verdant shore
    My infant footsteps trod;
'Twas there I learn'd to know and love
    The beauteous works of God.

In later years I've gazed upon
    Thy placid waves so bright;
Or mark'd them when stern winter's frosts
    Enchain'd them from the sight.

Or, when the angry storms have made
    Thy turbid waters rise,
I've silently admired the Power
    That rules thee from the skies.

And now my thoughts revert to thee,
    As far from thee I roam;
And mark, beside thy waves so free,
    That sacred spot—my home.

That home, where, a short time ago,
    I fondly bade adieu
Unto my earliest bosom friends,
    The dearest and most true.

There, too, within death's cold embrace,
  Where beauteous flowrets bloom,
Those whom I early loved and lost,
  Sleep in the silent tomb.

Then 'tis not strange that thou to me
  Shouldst ever seem most dear;
Or that my humble pen presumes
  To trace thy praises here.

For, should I roam o'er all the earth,
  I ne'er will find, I ween,
A fairer, sweeter spot to me,
  Than thou, my native stream.

PRACTISE WHAT YOU PREACH:
OR, EXAMPLE BETTER THAN PRECEPT.

Tell me not of garbled sermon,
   Elegance of thought and style;
Heard from out our modern pulpits
   Man from error to beguile.
Eloquence may charm the fancy,
   Summon an admiring crowd,
Who surround the gifted preacher
   With their praises, long and loud;
But if God's appointed servants
   Would their hearer's conscience reach,
Leading them in paths of wisdom—
   They must practise what they preach.

Parents, if your tender offspring
   Ye would lead in ways of truth,
Shielding them from the temptations
   That surround the path of youth;

Count as vain your time-worn maxims,
  And, to make your teaching sure,
Guide them—not alone by precept,
  But example, just and pure,
For, to shelter from the tempests
  Sin's dark clouds would cast 'round each
Tender flower of your protection,
  You must practise what you preach.

Teachers, if throughout your duties,
  Ever faithful you would be,
Not by words, but by your actions,
  Teach in all sincerity.
Youthful eyes are on you gazing,
  Youthful hearts your thoughts receive;
Eagerly they catch your accents,
  Eagerly your words believe;—
Then beware! lest by those actions,
  Untrue principles you teach;
And forget not you must ever
  Strive to practise what you preach.

Ye who would redeem a brother
  Through a Saviour's pard'ning love,
Know that by your bright example
  You must 'lure to joys above!

PRACTISE WHAT YOU PREACH.

Better were the world, and wiser,
    Full of goodness and of truth,
If, throughout each generation,
    Hoary age and buoyant youth,
All who preach the glorious gospel,
    All who govern, all who teach,
Would but learn this useful lesson—
    Always practise what you preach.

OMNISCIENCE.

"London makes mirth; but I know God hears
The sighs i' th' dark, and the dropping of tears.'
Gerald Massey.

How bless'd the thought, that on this nether sphere,
   That God who marks the tiny sparrow's fall,
Who gave existence unto all things here,
   His guardian care extendeth over all.

How bless'd for those astray from virtue's path,
   Pierc'd by the pois'nous arrows vice hath hurl'd,
And trembling 'neath high Heaven's impending wrath,
   Now mourn within the Londons of our world,

How bless'd for those who their good Father's home
   Have left, temptation's labyrinth to try;
As wand'rers and as outcasts doomed to roam—
   Weary of life, and yet afraid to die,

OMNISCIENCE.

To know when keenest anguish rends the heart,
    And untold grief finds vent alone in tears;
That e'en amid th' earth's remotest mart,
    The omnipresent One both sees and hears!

That One, who, veil'd in mortal flesh below,
    The weakness of that flesh Himself hath proved;
Meekly consenting that His blood should flow,
    To seal the pardon of the race He loved.

Earth's weary ones, behold your Sov'reign God!
    He reigns above in grace and mercy free;
In kindness doth He wield the chastening rod,
    Whispering—" Ye heavy-laden, come to me!"

What though your erring fellow-man, in scorn,
    Should pass you by upon the other side?—
Salvation points to that triumphant morn—
    The resurrection of the Crucified.

RANDOM THOUGHTS.

FOR THE NEW YEAR OF 1860.

LIGHTLY fall the crystal snow-flakes
   Over all the restless earth,
Like the down from angels' pinions,
Come they from those bright dominions.
Where, upon their ether pinions,
   Sail the clouds that gave them birth;
And they bear, amid their brightness,
Purity and virgin whiteness,
   Harbingers of winter's mirth.

Many eyes are on them gazing,
   As they softly fall around;
Many hearts are beating gladly,
Many pulses bounding madly,
Many, too, are throbbing sadly,

While hot tears bedew the ground;
For, for some, bright rays of gladness,
And for others, clouds of sadness,
  'Mid those shining flakes are found.

Votaries of wealth and fashion,
  As they mark those flakelets fall,
View them as some priceless treasure,
For they seem to them a measure,
Meting out its share of pleasure—
  Joy and pleasure unto all.
While the poor, upon them gazing,
And to Heav'n their eyes upraising,
  See them as a funeral pall.

For, to them, their silent language
  Tells of sternest want and woe;
Tells of cold and hunger pressing,
Tells of griefs, e'en more distressing,
Tells of anguish most oppressing,
  Known but to the poor below;
And to Him who careth for them,
Him whose love e'er watches o'er them,
  As they on their life-path go.

Thou who rulest storm and tempest,
   Life's dark conflicts and its cheer,
E'ër above the storm-cloud riding,
And for us with care providing,
To us, in Thy love abiding,
   Sanctify each hope and fear;
Till, enrob'd in snowy whiteness,
Our freed souls, in realms of brightness,
   Enter on a glad New Year.

THE INEBRIATE'S WIFE.

A PARODY.

Stay, husband—stay, and hear my woe!
   It is thy wife who kneels to thee;—
What thou art now, too well I know;
   And what thou wast, and what shouldst be.
To harshly chide I would forbear—
   My language shall be mild though sad:
Yet such neglect, from one so dear,
   Will drive me mad—will drive me mad!

King Alcohol hath chained thy soul—
   Hath bound it with resistless spell!
Dark is thy doom—thy destined goal!
   Oh, haste! That threat'ning fate dispel!
Oh, haste, my breaking heart to cheer!
   That breaking heart 'twill surely glad,
To know thou wilt no longer, here,
   Pursue a course so basely mad.

THE INEBRIATE'S WIFE.

He smiles in scorn and turns from me—
   Our hovel quits—I knelt in vain!
Hope's glimmering ray no more I see.
   'Tis gone—and all is gloom again.
Cold, bitter cold!—No warmth, no light!
   Life, all thy comforts once I had;
Yet, here I'm left this freezing night,
   By suff'ring driven almost mad.

'Tis sure some dream—some vision vain—
   What! I, the child of rank and wealth,
Am I the wretch endures this pain,
   'Reft of affection, friends, and health?
Ah! while I dwell on blessings fled,
   Which nevermore my heart shall glad,
How aches my heart, how burns my head—
   Such agony will drive me mad!

Hast thou, my child, forgot e'er this,
   A father's face—a father's tongue?
He has forgot your last fond kiss,
   Or 'round his neck how fast you clung;
Or how you sued for him to stay—
   How sternly he that suit forbade:
Or how—I'll drive such thoughts away—
   They'll make me mad—they'll make me mad!

His rosy lips once sweetly smiled—
   His mild blue eyes once brightly shone ;—
None ever bore a lovelier child—
   But ah! that loveliness has flown!
Flown—and I'll ne'er behold it more
   'Mid earthly scenes, my darling lad—
Thank God, thy suff'rings now are o'er,
   Else they had surely drove me mad.

Oh, hark! What mean those yells and cries?
   He home returns—the morning breaks—
He comes—I see his demon eyes—
   Now, now my inmost spirit quakes!
Help! help! He raves! O fearful woe!
   Such oaths to hear—such blasphemy!
My breath—my breath—I know—I know—
   From—anguish—soon—I shall—be free!

Yes, soon! For, lo you! while I speak,
   Seraphic strains I seem to hear—
Angelic hosts—your courts I seek ;—
   Joy—joy—the Father's throne I near!
Yet, unto Him one last fond prayer
   I'd breathe in heartfelt tones, though sad—
Him whom I love, Oh, spare—Oh, spare—
   Redeem—him—from—a course—so mad!

MY OTHER SELF.

Sometimes, methinks, I'm of two selves composed—
   The outer and the inner:
The inner prompts to high and noble deeds;
The outer acts; but ill, at best, succeeds,
   And seldom proves the winner;
Seldom attains that higher grade,
By worthier inner life portrayed;
And in life's general masquerade
   Seems always a beginner.

Could but the promptings of that inner self
   Be shown in pristine beauty,
Such words—such works 'twould to the world reveal,
As would in shadows of eclipse conceal
   All past attempts at duty;

Would charm the sight and inner sense,
With an acme of excellence
Known only to Omnipotence,
    In scenes of dazzling beauty.

And thus each day and hour I still endure
    This constant war internal—
The inner striving with the outer life,
And ne'er attaining, 'mid its earnest strife,
    Vict'ry o'er th' external.
Seldom, despite each prayer and tear,
Seeming to realize, while here,
A foretaste of that hallow'd sphere
    Of purest bliss eternal.

When one who heard unlawful words for man,
    Attained to the third heaven,
Lest too secure might grow his hope of bliss
In worlds to come, a "thorn of flesh," in this,
    To him was wisely given;
And when he prayed it might removed be,
The answer came—"Sufficient unto thee
My grace both now and evermore shall be,
    Till Life's frail cord is riven!"

Then shun thou not, aspiring inner self,
  This war of flesh with spirit!
God's sov'reign grace to all sufficient proves;
In mercy ever chastening whom He loves;
  The measure of thy merit
Shall not escape His righteous view;
And if thou faithful prove, and true,
Ever thy own appointed due
  Thou shalt inherit.

OUR FATHER.

"The world has been thousands of years, and not yet learned the first two words of the Lord's prayer; and not until all tribes and nations have learned these, will His kingdom come, and His will be done on earth, as it is in heaven."—*H. B. Stowe.*

"Our Father!" Name by childhood breathed
    Around the homestead hearth!
The guardian kind, whose care defends
    That sacred spot of earth.

"Our Father!" Thus the Saviour prayed!
    Thus He taught us to pray,
When asking of our heavenly Guide
    Our "daily bread each day."

"Our Father!" Words unheeded oft!
    Yet, did we own their power,
'Twould keep the soul's dread foes at bay
    In dark temptation's hour.

"Our Father!" Teach us thus to pray,
  When angry passions burn
Within our hearts, for injuries
  They'd prompt us to return!

"Our Father!" Let us not forget
  How strong that sacred tie,
When a neglected brother claims
  Our active sympathy!

"Our Father!" Let us learn their worth!
  For never, until then,
Can we e'er realize on earth
  Peace and good will to men.

THE WRECK OF A BROKEN LIFE.

METHOUGHT I stood upon life's ocean strand,
And mark'd a helpless object, far from land,
   Amid its angry strife;
Rudely the billows heav'd it to and fro;
The wreck, of all wrecks direst here below—
   That of a broken life.

I saw it in the swelling surges toss'd;
With shatter'd masts, torn sails, and rudder lost—
   Daring the briny foam;
I saw it striving on its dangerous way,
To seek the entrance of some port or bay
   That might conduct it home.

No cheering pharos warn'd from danger dread;
All human aid had fail'd—all hope had fled
   In any earthly power;
But still it struggled;—striving yet to save
Itself from death beneath the foaming wave,
   In that dark, threat'ning hour.

All vain the strife—its fury would not cease;
No waken'd sleeper yet had murmur'd—" Peace!"
   That Sleeper, still uncall'd,
Could not befriend in that portentous hour,
Because the struggling victim spurn'd His power,
   Though dangers dire appall'd.

Then I discern'd, upon the billows high,
The Ark of Safety riding fearlessly—
   Its Pilot at the helm;
That dauntless Pilot, that unerring Guide,
Who can protect against whatever tide
   May threaten to o'erwhelm.

And then, methought, that wreck He yearn'd to bless,
Rais'd timidly its signal of distress,
   And rais'd it not in vain;
For soon, within the Ark His strong arm drew
That sinking wreck; rebuk'd, and whisper'd, too,
   " Peace to the angry main!"

That Sleeper and that Pilot both are one;
They bear the rescued now securely on
   Toward an eternal shore;
In vain the storms arise—the tempests blow;
'Neath His protection it no fear can know;
   Its perils all are o'er.

Ye broken life-wrecks, with a care as true,
The same unerring Pilot waits for you;
   Waits to convey you home;
Fear not to enter His all-saving Ark;
That Ark protects from ev'ry tempest dark—
   Each danger that may come.

WHITE SWEARING.

There is a legend, old, and quaint, and rustic,
  A legend of a lad,
Who, taking once his airy flight through dream-land,
  This curious vision had:

He dream'd that he had died and gone to judgment;
  And that with him did come
All th' unnumber'd hosts of earth and heaven,
  To hear their final doom.

And one was there, arraigned for white-lying;
  Or telling lies in jest;
Who on the left was plac'd—'mongst other culprits,
  When past the solemn test.

This was a dream—yet I have often wonder'd
  If such the fate must be
Of the white-liar, what shall the white-swearer
  In other regions see?

Some "goody-good folks," who would shrink and
    shudder,
  A real oath to hear,
Seem to indulge the practice of white-swearing,
  Untrammell'd by a fear.

They swear by slamming doors and throwing objects
  That happen in their way;
They swear by modest little oaths, invented
  For Christians (?) such as they.

Can the same fount hold waters sweet and bitter?
  Not readily, I ween!
Then look you to the source from whence proceedeth
  Such outbursts of the spleen!

I do not wish to meddle or be curious,
  But can't help wondering here—
What is the penalty, when for white-swearing
  The guilty must appear.

INDEPENDENCE MUST HAVE LIMITS.

"Independence must have limits!"
   Says the caviller at right—
"Lay aside your sword and helmet!
   Cease to don your armor bright!
Combats, carried to excesses,
   Never yet did any good;—
Seek not to obtain redresses,
   E'en at cost of your heart's blood!
Guard ye well each daring action!
   Guard ye each undaunted word!
Guard them! lest in feeling's fountain
   Bitter draughts ye may have stirred."

Independence must have limits!
   Was it thus our father's taught?
Was it such a Declaration
   They to England's sov'reign brought?
Prompted by this cowardly motto,
   Struggled they for liberty?

Did they by such half-way prowess,
  Vanquish Britain's tyranny?
No! their Stoic independence
  Proudly spurned such cringing laws—
Fortunes, lives, and sacred honor—
  All they pledged in Freedom's cause.

Independence must have limits!
  Yes! when Error's reign is o'er;
When fair Truth, by her untrammell'd,
  Rises to be crushed no more;
When, like disembodied spirits,
  Suffering humanity
From all outrage and oppression
  Boasts herself forever free;
When no more, o'er earth and ocean,
  Contumely's war trumpet sounds;—
Then, and not until that moment,
  Independence may have bounds.

THE EXODUS OF THE NINETEENTH CENTURY.

"The exodus of the slave will be through the Red Sea."—*Lovejoy.*

BLOOD! blood! blood!
   How flows that crimson tide!
Oh, when will the sources that swell its streams
   E'er cease to be supplied?
Must perish another "Pharaoh's host,"
In its terrible depths thus fiercely toss'd,
While "Israel's oppress'd" on dry land are cross'd?
   Blood! blood! blood!

Groans! groans! groans!
   How they load th' ambient air!
While ascends to heaven's eternal throne
   Each agonizing prayer!
For eighty years have such groans been heard;
Such bitter groans from our South-land pour'd,
Yet Columbia's bosom was scarcely stirr'd!
   Groans! groans! groans!

Death! death! death!
   What fearful numbers fall!
When to Adam's enslaved a ransom came,
   One Life atoned for all!
Then must so many loved be lost—
So many thresholds by sorrow cross'd,
Ere our nation redeems what her crime has cost?
   Death! death! death!

Grief! grief! grief!
   List to those deep-drawn sighs!
North, South, East, West—in war-drear'd homes,
   Successively they rise!
Such grief, such tears have long been known
In cotton-fields—in rice-swamps lone ;—
Now from Afric's to Europe's race they've flown!
   Grief! grief! grief!

Tears! tears! tears!
   How copiously they flow!
Wrung from heart-depths, their founts are stirr'd
   By keenest mental woe!
Baptized in blood and tears, our land
In future years, may firmer stand,
Chasten'd by an avenging Hand!
   Tears! tears! tears!

Light! light! light!
  It breaks through darkest gloom!
It pledges America's enslaved
  Freedom in Freedom's home!
Author of light! oh, bless that ray!
Guide it upon its heavenward way,
Till it attains to perfect day!
  Light! light! light!

IN MEMORIAM.

Died, at Fortress Monroe, Va., of Typhoid Fever, on the 18th of 1st month, 1862, in the 25th year of his age, Dr. Chas. K. Thomas, of 11th Pa. Cavalry.—At Camp Pierpont, Va., 1st month, 28th, 1862, in the 19th year of his age, of Brain Fever, Benj. H. Roberts, of the 4th Reg. Penna. Reserves.—At Hilton Head, Port Royal, S. C., on the 30th of 1st month, of Typhoid Fever, Sergeant Gerritt S. Hambleton, of the 97th Reg. P. V., aged 22 years.

> Give thanks
> That they are safe with Him who hath the power
> O'er pain and sin and death.—*L. H. Sigourney.*

PEACEFULLY they slumber now!
   Peaceful, 'neath the valley's clod!
Pallid, cold, each manly brown!
   Priceless spirits gone to God.
From the camp's excitement free,
   From its dangers and its toils,
In celestial liberty,
   Safe from all the Tempter's foils.

IN MEMORIAM.

'Twas not theirs to do and dare
  On the gory battle-plain;
'Twas not theirs to perish where
  Thousands of the brave are slain.
But did they less truly die
  In their country's righteous cause,
Answering her earnest cry,
  Aiding to sustain her laws?

Was the sacrifice less great,
  They upon her altar laid,
Than the heroes who in state
  Wait a nation's homage paid?
Ask the stricken mourners left
  Weeping for their early dead!
Ask the circles thus bereft
  Of their brilliant "earth-stars" fled!

Ask our country's future good
  When hostilities shall cease;
And her noblest brotherhood
  Hail with joy the dawn of peace!
Costly treasures these to yield!
  Worthy of the richest gain!
May the forum and the field
  Prove them yielded not in vain!

AFTER THE BATTLE.

The smoke-cloud is merged in the pure ether sea,
  And hushed the artillery's rattle;
And Luna looks down with a face calmly pale,
  On the gory field after the battle.
Low, low on the clayey bed, red with their blood,
  Friend and foe, horse and rider are lying;
While e'er and anon, a heart-rending groan
  Tells the fate of the wounded and dying.

On Fancy's light wing let us soar o'er that spot
  Renown'd in Columbia's story;
Let us gaze for a while on that carnage which shows
  Her record of shame and of glory!
Let us muse on each scene which the moonlight reveals!
  Scenes that make the heroic heart tremble;
Scenes that waken the deep fount of feeling within—
  Such feeling we would not dissemble.

AFTER THE BATTLE.

Here lies one with a miniature 'neath his cold hand,
    Of a lovely and beautiful woman ;—
Did his warrior's heart love that being in life,
    With a fervor the deepest that's human?
Was that prototype loving friend, sister, or wife?
    (Too youthful it seems for his mother);
These myst'ries we never may know in this life:
    They await the pure light of another.

And here, with his Bible worn close to his breast,
    Another in silence reposes;
That Bible—few words might the history tell,
    Which e'en now it in silence discloses.
'Twas the gift of his mother—her last, parting gift,
    Which she bade him to love and to cherish;
And that treasure he bore as he bravely went forth
    The foremost in battle to perish.

Here are two; in death's slumber they rest side by side;
    Yet no contrast could e'er have been greater;
For one is enrob'd in a patriot's garb,
    The other the garb of a traitor.
Why is this? Was the conflict so fearful that thus
    In mutual embrace they have perished?
Or did mem'ry recall a friendship, that e'en
    'Mid rebellion and strife had not perished.

And this, this is war! such as fair Avon's bard,
   So famed in poetical story,
In language of pathos hath made to possess
   Pomp, circumstance, undying glory.
God spare our loved country more glory like this!
   From such circumstance, pomp, e'er defend her!
And instead, the bright ensigns of Freedom and
     Peace
   Sustain in their unfading splendor.

NAVIS REPUBLICÆ.

Navis Republicæ! Why sails she now,
Shatter'd her timbers all, from stern to prow?
Stormy the sea she plows, low'ring her sky?
Hanging portentous clouds o'er her on high?
Who's her commander now? Who are her crew?
Are they not brave as wont, faithful and true?
Where are her Jeffersons, Franklins, and Lees?
Carrolls of Carrollton? Are none of these
Near her to succor her ere she shall wreck?
Whence comes yon pirate crew, thronging her deck?
Blood is upon that deck—blood stains each wave
That 'gainst her creaking keel madly doth lave!
Ha! still her banner waves! See I aright?—
Pierc'd through with bullet-holes! Ah! what a sight—
Grieving my spirit thus!—Mount Vernon's son,
Navis, such fate for thee ne'er would have known;
Tell me what foreign foe dar'd to assail
Thus our loved "stars and stripes," braving the gale?

Navis Republicæ! Her signal bell
Rings out the solemn words—" All is not well!"
Yet, "Pater Patræ," no foreign foe
Dealt on our ensign proud that cowardly blow;
Pierc'd it with bullet-holes;—Mount Vernon's heir—
Sire—thine own flesh and blood helped place them
    there;
Treason hath madden'd them—made their hearts
    cold;
Summon'd in serried ranks Arnolds of old;
Forth from protection strong madly they've flown,
Built in a frenzied hour craft of their own;—
Raised amid pond'rous masts their "stars and bars;"
Taunted insultingly our "stripes and stars."
Vainly our Middletons, Hancocks, Treat Paines,
Prescotts and Sullivans, Putnams and Waynes,
Rise in defence of her, manning each post,
Vowing their gallant ship shall not be lost.
Spirit of Washington, patriot sire,
Tell us, while dimly burns Liberty's fire,
Why gains each leak so fast? Can nothing save?
Must our storm-shatter'd barque sink 'neath the
    wave?

Navis Republicæ! In days of yore
Was it for this we such sacrifice bore?

All that was dearest pledged—all to sustain
Thee, our own fragile barque, daring the main?
Strong hast thou grown since then—what means this
    strife?—
Homicide—Fratricide threat'ning thy life?
Ha! Now I see it all! Now I behold!
Mark ye yon dusky forms crowding her hold!
Panting for liberty—Heaven's free air!
Think ye to save the ship while they are there?
Shame, shame upon you all! Do ye not know
Crime such as this can't avert Heaven's blow?
Quick!—Cast the life-boats forth into the sea!
Bid all take refuge there who would be free!
Give them their "turn at pump," aiding to save
Ere your tossed vessel is lost 'neath the wave!
Sad was the oversight, barque of the free,
When such a heritage left we to thee.
Ha! they're obeying now! Captain, well done!
Now may thy vessel move fearlessly on,
Purging iniquity, cleansing each stain—
Claiming God's blessing forever. Amen!

WHEN THE WAR ENDS.

When this bloody war is ended,
   When this sanguine strife is o'er,
When the din and shock of battle
   Through our land resounds no more;
When dethroned, foul-hearted Treason
   Fills an ignominious tomb;
And the hordes that raised his banner
   Justly meet a traitor's doom,
Will there be throughout our nation,
   One blest home from anguish free?
Anguish caused by mad rebellion,
   And inhuman butchery;
One fond heart unscathed by sorrow,
   One bright eye, undimmed by tears;
Tears shed for some slain beloved one,
   Sacrificed in manhood's years?

WHEN THE WAR ENDS.

" When the war ends "—writes the soldier
    To his cherished friends and home ;
" When, through Slavery's dominions
    'Tis no more my lot to roam ;
When my country's call is answered,
    When her victories are won ;
And the dawn of peace proclaimeth
    That th' warrior's task is done ;
Then to home's alluring precincts,
    Trust I safely to return,
Joying that throughout our nation
    Freedom's watch-fires brightly burn."
Hopeful words!—Words fitly spoken
    By the loyal-hearted brave !
But how often hushed to silence
    In a laurell'd hero's grave.

When this cruel war is ended,
    When its horrid scenes are o'er,
Blushingly, my mother country,
    Blushingly wilt thou deplore
That, within thy truthful annals
    Thou a record must retain
Of a crime so dark and damning
    Nought but blood could cleanse the stain ;

That, in fratricidal conflict,
    Fiercely, desperately strove
Sons whom thy fond bosom nurtur'd—
    Sons who shared thy common love;
That against thy star-gemmed banner,
    All ungratefully arose
Arms that should for aye have shielded
    That proud ensign from its foes.

When the war ends—who can tell us
    When and where that end shall be?
Heaven decrees its termination—
    UNIVERSAL LIBERTY!
Freemen, will ye dare to falter
    Till that high decree's fulfilled?
If ye dare, then worse than vainly
    Has your precious blood been spilled!
Worse than vainly, friends and kindred,
    Mothers, sisters, daughters, wives,
Mourn ye those who in this contest,
    Bravely, freely, yield their lives.
Choose to-day then!—Choose between them,
    Whom to serve!—Who is your Lord?
Choose ye Baal?—Share his curses!
    Choose ye God?—His high rewards!

FORT PILLOW.

"For the devil is come down unto you, having great wrath, because he knoweth that he hath but a short time."—*Rev.* xii. 12.

MOURNFUL tidings from our borders! Mournful tidings from the West!
Tidings of the cowardly slaughter of our bravest and our best!
Draping the dark pall of sorrow over homesteads richly blest.

Mournful tidings! Ah, how mournful! when our shrinking mental sight
Marks, in all their ghastly horror, in their soul-appalling might,
Visions of the charred and mangled victims of that treach'rous fight.

Happy omen of thy future, shattered, suff'ring country mine,
Omen of a purer freedom proffered unto thee and
 thine—
Seek ye, sinful generation, for a more propitious
 sign?

See ye not on yon dark war-cloud, even now, the
 arching bow,
Pledging us the speedy triumph of Rebellion's over-
 throw?
Triumph o'er the craven spirit that can scourge a
 fallen foe.

See ye not the cast-out demon, writhing, foaming in
 its wrath,
Maddened by its desperation, deeply conscious that
 it hath
But a short time yet to linger in its dang'rous, down-
 ward path?

Patience, then, ye toiling millions! Pray for patience once again!
Though still louder clank the fetters of Oppression's
 galling chain—
Patience! for that louder clanking marks their sever-
 ing in twain.

Heaven knows what ye have suffered! Heaven will
 the crime avenge—
Conscious that these darksome moments but foretell
 a brighter change,
Grant we to our erring brother rather pity than
 revenge.

Heaven knows what ye have suffered! Only
 Heaven now doth know
What we're destined all to suffer, ere is dealt the
 final blow,
Hurling to its sure destruction, this, our direst, deadliest foe.

But that blow will fall as surely as a just God reigns
 above—
Chastened then, but not despairing, let us wait the
 hour to prove
That these Fatherly corrections all contain a Father's
 love.

OUR DEAD HEROES.

" They never fail who die in a good cause."

I COME not now to tell the mournful story
   Of the renowned and nation-honored dead;
Who, in th' acme of their fame and glory,
   In Freedom's cause have bled.

All honor to the vet'rans, loyal, fearless,
   Whose lives within our country's shrine are lain;
Who, with undaunted prowess, truly peerless,
   Led forth her martial train.

More gifted pens unite to do them rev'rence,
   More able voices join in notes of praise;
I would not then aspire, amid such cadence,
   To swell my humble lays.

Mine be the task to chant, in dirge-like numbers,
   A requiem for th' unlauded brave—
The humbler hero, who now calmly slumbers
   In some unnoticed grave.

Some peaceful sleeper 'neath the restless waters
  Of a famed river, creek, or surging bay;
Mourn'd by fond sisters, mother, wife, or daughters,
  In homes, far, far away.

Some patient sufferer in rebel prison,
  In Fed'ral hospital, or fort, or camp;—
Whose fervent prayers for Truth's advance have risen,
  As wan'd life's flickering lamp.

Some wounded champion on the field of battle,
  Falling unheeded 'mid the carnage dread;
And moaning out, unheard, the drear death-rattle
  Upon his gory bed.

Or some lone picket, faithful to his duty,
  Treading in silence his appointed round;
Musing on home-scenes love has clothed in beauty;
  Till, on death's mission bound,

A fatal bullet from a rebel weapon,
  Gleaming like lightning through the mid-night gloom,
Dissolves his faith-illumined visions halcyon,
  In sight beyond the tomb.

Braves such as these, are daily, hourly falling;
　Their eulogies unsung, their names unknown;
Their blood, like righteous Abel's, loudly calling
　Unto Jehovah's throne.

For them my pen would trace these dirge-like measures,
　For them my soul in sympathy would burn
With 'reft ones, mourning for their household treasures,
　That nevermore return.

Such are the gems, my loved, but guilty nation,
　From fond and yearning hearts remorseless torn,
To pay the price of thy regeneration,
　Thy second natal morn.

Thy infant life in pristine freshness glowing,
　By blood and tears its advent mark'd on earth;—
Blood, blood and tears the advent are foreshowing,
　Of this, thy purer birth.

In Adam thou hast died; in Christ reviving,
　Go forth triumphant on thy heavenward way!
Incessantly 'gainst sin and evil striving,
　Press on to perfect day!

Thou shouldst "love much ;" for great has been thy
    error—
Chasten'd by this severe internal strife ;
Emerging from this Modern " Reign of Terror,"
    Live thou a truer life !

WHAT I SAW, HEARD, AND THOUGHT,

AT THE THIRD ANTI-SLAVERY DECADE HELD IN CONCERT HALL, PHILADA., DECEMBER 3d and 4th, 1863.

This is the place—the hall where many a scene
Like to the present has enacted been;
But not in times like these—for thirty years
These champions for truth, 'mid taunts and jeers,
'Mid persecutions, scoffs, and proud disdain,
Hoping 'gainst hope, yet deeming nothing vain
That might promote the cause they had espoused,
Or thwart the demon that their zeal aroused—
Have firmly stood—a small, but dauntless band,
Pledged to the right, united, heart and hand,
'Gainst the foul crime polluting all our land.
 Careless spectators oft the scene surveyed,
Idly regretting, needlessly dismayed
By the loud clamor opposition made.

While some, like me, with zealous ardor fired,
Have stood aloof, and silently admired.
Have stood aloof! been silent! And for why?
Not from a lack of kindred sympathy;
Though time there was—with shame I it confess—
When I discerned not Christ's true righteousness
In aught of this. In early life 'twas thus,
False education made me what I was;—
But later years, thank God, a change have wrought;
All prejudice o'ercome, I now am brought
To sit with them as one in feeling, thought.
I've stood aloof, been silent, but for this—
A painful sense of my unworthiness;
My own unfitness for so great a task;
And though I now most gladly doff the mask
That long has screened me, I'd be silent still—
Content to manifest my ready will
To sit and listen as each speaker's voice
Salutes my ear; and inwardly rejoice
That right at last has triumphed over might—
That morn has dawned after so dark a night.
And mine is not the only heart thus changed,
That long has been an alien and estranged
From truth's great sheep-fold. Mark ye not around
What order reigns? What interest profound

Enwraps the throng, save when prolonged applause
Salutes some earnest champion of the cause?
   What's wrought the change? From Sumter's war-
      scathed walls
The answer comes. In thunder-tones it falls
On startled ears—"They who refuse to hear
The voice of justice when the sky is clear,
'Mid blood and carnage shall that voice revere!"
   The morning session's o'er, else I might tell
How on my ears the written message fell,
Of him, "The Quaker Bard of Amesbury,"
And other advocates of liberty;
But I'll content me with what's yet to be.
What objects meet my gaze? Upon yon stand,
An auction-block for slaves—bane of our land—
Is brought to view! What stories it might tell
Of grief and horror! But I may not dwell
Upon them now. One of more just renown—
A life-like portrait of the martyr, Brown—
Hangs just beyond it. 'Tis a happy thought
That thus in close proximity has brought,
As if by contrast, objects so remote
In worth and meaning—bidding us denote
That mute memento of past woe and crime,
And this, of deeds heroic and sublime.

A voice is heard; and one whose worthy name
Has long been coupled with abuse and blame—
Columbia's children, be it to your shame!—
Returning good for evil in this hour
When his loved cause is gaining strength and power,
Slav'ry's undaunted foe, Lloyd Garrison,
Welcomes the audience in kindest tone.

A speaker he announces—List to him!
Of unpretending name—J. M. McKim!
Yet at that name the hearts of millions thrill!
Hear him as he relates how, through God's will,
He has been led into the path he treads,
Thus showering blessings on the humblest heads.
Within his voice how much of kindness reigns!
And yet, methinks, his speech a fault contains;
I'd tell it here—a little cloud he names
This mighty movement 'gainst oppression's aims,
Not larger in the past than human hand,
And spreading now abroad o'er all the land.
I'd rather he had said—The glimm'ring light
Which now is growing brighter and more bright;
For see! The clouds are all dispelling now,
'Mid war's loud thunders; while, on Freedom's brow
A brighter halo and a more divine
Than e'er was hers must in the future shine.

Footsteps resound along the spacious aisle,
The speaker's earnest tones are hushed a while,
As pass, with measured tread, a retinue
Of sable forms arrayed in army blue;
A delegation from Camp Wm. Penn,
Under command of Sergeant Brown—brave men!
A welcome they receive on ev'ry hand,
As they advance; upon the speaker's stand
Are seats prepared for that heroic band.
While o'er their heads that ensign's colors blend,
Which they have sworn to die or to defend.
Tears dim my eyes—tears from the inward strife
Caused by this foretaste of celestial life;
A life where caste and color are unknown,
Save as a unit 'round the "Great White Throne."

Another name's announced—and Mary Grew,
One of the faithful, patient, toiling few
Who've borne their weary burden in the heat
Comes forth with brief but earnest words, to greet
Each eager list'ner; and contrast this hour
With that in which our subtle foe had power.

Anon another one—Samuel J. May;
A Reverend he is termed, and yet, how gay,
How full of wit and merriment doth seem
His words and manner for so grave a theme;

But mark you, 'neath that sparkling eloquence
An under-current flows—a consciousness
Of the great burden 'tis his lot to bear,
Responsibilities 'tis his to share;
Yet mingling it with mirth—we'll trust him, then,
As far, and farther than some graver men.

Now comes forth one—ne'er let her be forgot—
That vet'ran in the cause—Lucretia Mott;
From youth to age, e'er faithful to the right,
To the true guidance of the "inner light,"
Clad in her modest Quaker garb, she seems
Like some chaste spirit one beholds in dreams.
Hear her, as with deep pathos she doth tell
Each sad experience; and anon doth dwell
On scenes more ludicrous in by-gone years,
Exciting in their turn both mirth and tears;—
Enlisting ev'ry heart in the good cause,
She takes her seat amid prolonged applause.

The morning dawns! And yet its dawnings bright
Hide not the radiance of another light
Upon Truth's watchtower—modest though its mien,
As H. Ward Beecher comes upon the scene.
His words are few; yet fraught with weight and
    power;
A world-acknowleged champion for this hour,

When light and darkness, in a bloody strife,
Hold in their hands our nation's death or life.
Blessings upon him! Aye, and God will bless
Such faithful teachers of his righteousness.

Next Chas. C. Burleigh's deep-toned voice is heard;
Is there a soul within its sound not stirred
By its pure eloquence? A heart not fired
With the true zeal his language has inspired?

But I must haste me! Speakers multiply
Upon me here, and I must pass them by;
Save but to note the names of Anthony,
The Fosters, Powell, Wagner, Stone, and she,
One of the noblest women of her age—
The Freedman's earnest helper—F. D. Gage.
And Johnson, too, whose editorial pen
And fluent tongue so oft have claimed for men
Rights, equal rights, their God-appointed due,
Whatever be their nation, clime, or hue.

The evening session—See! an alien stands
Upon the platform—not from foreign lands;
But alienated by a tainted blood
That man's weak judgment has pronounced not good!
'Tis Robert Purvis! Though his words are few,
They mark the gentleman, the patriot true;
Asking that God a country yet may save,
Who ne'er to him and his protection gave.

Now Tilton's voice is heard; one young in years,
But old in wisdom, on the stage appears;
Mark ye that manly face, whose poet soul
Illumes each lineament, seems to control
His ev'ry word and act! How brilliantly
His burning words, denouncing slavery,
Sparkle with gems of truth and poesy!
Another still from 'mongst the good and great,
Senator Wilson of the old " Bay State,"
In Congress halls e'er true to Freedom's cause,
Rises 'mid rounds of deafening applause;
A statesman's logic it is his to wield,
Adapted more to forum than to field;
And savoring much of practical good sense,
Destined to win a nation's confidence.
Next Douglass stands—a living monument
Of what man dare do, when his soul is rent
By tortures wrought on his clay tenement.
Enough of Southern fire his speech contains,
Enough of Afric's blood flows through his veins
To make impressive, while it entertains,
His speech, gesticulation. Spoke he, then,
A sentence; I would name it here again;—
"The day, the hour is not yet passed," said he,
In which is coupled much of infamy

With him, the true and tried philanthropist,
The scorned, world-hated Abolitionist."
Thanks, dusky orator, those words of thine
Have proved consoling to this soul of mine;—
Then I am not the sneaking coward I thought,
Seeking, at this late hour, where long have wrought
These earnest, faithful laborers in the sun,
A tranquil entrance when the work is done;
Thanks, thanks to thee! I gladly now will share
Whate'er of scorn, reproach, 'tis yours to bear;
Joying that I'm thought worthy with the rest,
To suffer and endure for Christ's oppressed.

 Anon, another voice salutes my ear,
And Annie Dickinson's clear tones I hear;
That fearless one, whose touching eloquence
Has won for her a path to eminence.
Both to her sex, and to her country true,
Answering the question—"What can woman do?"
She closes; could not found a brighter goal,
This feast of reason, and this flow of soul.

 I leave this scene with feelings of regret;
One which, while life endures, I'll not forget;
For, whate'er pleasures yet my lot befall,
Methinks I'll ever place above them all,
My intellectual feast in Concert Hall.

FROM GETTYSBURG.

"There's the carrier, Lottie! The news of to-day
He's bringing! Then, haste, lay your sewing away,
And read to me, darling! You know that my sight
Is failing; and since, in the mansions of light
Your mother awaits us; and Edward has gone
A warrior for freedom, our home had seemed lone,
But for you, gentle daughter, whose duties, well borne,
Have enlivened the gloom that it else might have worn.
Then read to me, darling! You're all I've left, now,
To smooth the deep furrows care leaves on my brow.
Have Vicksburg, Port Hudson, surrendered? And say!—
How progresses the war in the 'Keystone' to-day?

Is Lee's army vanquish'd? Are his hordes driven
    back?
Or are rebel invaders still scenting our track?
You're silent—you're pale—does the news give you
    pain!"—
"Dearest father, I fear brother Edward is slain!
Here's his regiment—name—aye, 'tis certainly he!
He was second lieutenant of Company C."
"Great Father, have pity!—My brave, noble boy,
Once the pride of my heart, once a fond mother's
    joy—
Is he in the vigor of manhood laid low
By the murderous fire of a traitorous foe?
Must he silently rest' neath the valley's cold clod—
A martyr to freedom, to truth, and to God?
His mother, perchance—but, no! I'll not say
What she might have done, had she lived till the
    day
When he asked for permission to join in the strife
'Gainst the poison—the bane of our national life—
I fought under Perry—then could I forbear
To grant the consent that he asked? Could I dare
To restrain his young feet from the path that I trod?
No! I gave him to Liberty—gave him to God!

My off'ring's accepted ; then why should I crave
To possess it again? I'll be brave! I'll be brave!
For us is the suff'ring, for him the relief!
Then how vain is our sorrow! how selfish our
    grief!
The Union star brightens—then, though he be slain,
His precious young life-blood was not shed in vain!
Dear Lottie, I'm trembling—I'm cold—and my sight
Grows dim and yet dimmer—a marvellous light
Greets my vision internal—my wife—and my son."—
Christ shield thee, young mourner, so fragile and
    lone!
Christ shield thee, and all who like thee hourly
    mourn
The lŏv'd ones who've reach'd the mysterious
    bourne!
Ah, well! 'tis but brief! When life's burden's laid
    down,
The more pond'rous the cross the more glitt'ring the
    crown ;
And martyrs for truth shall eternally stand
With the blood-ransom'd throng at Jehovah's right
    hand."

STRENGTH THROUGH ADVERSITY.

> "Strong grows the oak in the sweeping storm;
> Safely the flower sleeps under the snow;
> And the farmer's hearth is never warm,
> Till the cold winds start to blow."
>
> *Holland's Bitter Sweet.*

HEIR to a boon immortal—fellow heir,
   Some words of kindly cheer I'd proffer thee;
Would seek thy spirit in communion, where
   It may seek mine—in kindred sympathy.
Hast thou ne'er felt, when anguish ruled the hour,
   And life seem'd weary, lonely, dark, and drear;
A want of trust in an Omniscient Power,
   A vague uncertainty, a nameless fear,
A wav'ring faith in Him, the Ruler of our sphere?

Stung with ingratitude, in spirit crush'd,
   When foes have triumph'd, and when friends have failed;
When vice o'er virtue stood with victory flush'd,
   And might 'gainst right on ev'ry side prevail'd;

When, one by one, thy fondest aims o'erthrown,
  Each earthly hope and aspiration died;
Within thy heart-depths hast thou never known
  A deep'ning interest in the True and Tried?
A yearning, yet a dread to seek the Crucfied?

I, too, have trod that path; I, too, have felt
  That inward shrinking from the dread unknown;
Yearn'd for the confidence of those who knelt
  In humble faith before the Father's throne.
I, too, have falter'd in my pilgrim course,
  When life's frail bubbles in my grasp have broke;
When Jove's just chastenings have wrought remorse;
  And I have bow'd and thank'd Him for the stroke;
Have found His burden light; joy'd in His easy yoke.

Have known my faith grow strong amid the storm;
  Have found hope's blossoms safe beneath the snow;
Have felt my soul's recesses grow more warm,
  When cold and adverse winds relentless blow;
Freely, Jehovah says, as ye receive,
  Freely dispense unto your fellow-men,
Such gifts, such blessings as can best relieve
  The doubting spirit in its sojourn, when,
A wanderer from home, it would return again.

And, as a traveller, who bewilder'd treads
   Lone and benighted o'er an unknown way;
When young Aurora her bright mantle spreads,
   Shedding abroad the dawning light of day;
Essays to cheer his fellow pilgrims o'er
     The dangerous pathway he himself hath trod;—
Sojourning traveller toward the peaceful shore,
   The pure, celestial city of our God—
So would I solace thee in the dark path I've trod.

Dost thou e'er tremble when the pall, the bier
   Wake in thy bosom visions of the hour
That brings to thee the end of all things here?
   When in the presence of unerring Power
Thy soul shall stand, 'reft of its earthly clay?—
     Tremble no more! 'Tis better far for thee,
When dawns at last that sure and final day,
   At a Divine than human bar to be;—
Judged by a Sov'reign, just, and full of sympathy.

That Sov'reign knows the willing spirit's strife,
   When the weak flesh would bid that spirit stray;
Directs its upward course from death to life,
   And guides its progress in the narrow way;

And He will lead that willing spirit forth,
  When transient earthly scenes dissolve from sight;
Freely vouchsafe the measure of its worth,
  And merge in glory of celestial light
The darkness that so oft hath gloom'd our mental night.

And there is darkness brooding o'er our land;
  A darkness that oft threatens to o'erwhelm;
A darkness that its fearful reign began,
  Almost coeval with our infant realm;
Its shades, extending with our nation's growth,
  Threw 'round her vitals a resistless spell;
To yield its hideous power seem'd ever loath;
  At Sumter sought to toll her funeral knell,
And more portentous grew when brave young Ellsworth fell.

Its shadows broaden'd; and its haughty crest
  Rose high; when, marshalling his valiant train,
The "lion-hearted" champion of the West
  Yielded his life on Springfield's battle-plain.
It drap'd our Senate-halls in deepest gloom;
  It hush'd therein a voice of eloquence;
And oped again the portals of the tomb,
  When Broderick's eulogist was summon'd hence,
Sharing alike a nation's love and confidence.

Its pall grows blacker as we journey on
   Through the Red Sea of fratricidal blood;
As our best, noblest patriots, one by one,
   From their heart-fountains swell the crimson flood.
But has this darkness, have these adverse gales,
   These dire Aceldamas throughout our land
Our inner life impair'd? As each assails,
   Do we grow strong when we as victors stand?
Or when some rude repulse has met our warrior
   band?

Did we gain strength when Burnside's gallant corps
   The serried ranks of traitorous New Berne broke?
Or mark'd our cherish'd colors floating o'er
   The sea-girt shores of rebel Roanoke?
Did we gain strength when Donelson's dread scenes
   Echoed glad shouts on its redemption day?
Did we gain strength when crescent New Orleans
   Almost resistless yielded to our sway,
And the glad tidings sped upon their joyous way?

Ah, no! relying on an arm of flesh,
   Proud "Worldly Wisdom" then presum'd to see
Our martial thousands soon returning fresh
   From battle-fields elate with victory.

Visions of a re-union like the past,
  Danc'd, gaily danc'd before enamor'd eyes;
Peace on a basis that could never last;
  A retrograde; a cowardly compromise
'Gainst liberty, that boon all honest patriots prize.

'Twas not in hours like these we stronger grew;
  For then the Tempter was alluring us
To substitute the old wine for the new;
  Error for truth; and sin for righteousness.
'Twas when, o'erwhelmed by Richmond's crimson
    tide,
  Our decimated army sought retreat;
When, dauntless still, they to Antietam hied,
  A desperate, aggressive foe to meet,
'Mid scenes with carnage, woe, and misery replete.

When once again Manassas' bloody ground
  Was fiercely trod by a contending host;
When once again the cannon's booming sound
  Proclaim'd the fearful truth—" a battle lost!"
When death, disaster, on all sides appall,
  And loyal bosoms were by anguish torn;
When suff'ring wounded to our Capitol,
  Mangled and bleeding, were by hundreds borne—
Then came our strength; dawn'd our salvation morn.

'Twas then, and not till then, our Chieftain dar'd
  To issue that Immortal Document,
For whose existence anxious hearts have shar'd
  In fervent prayer; and whose wise intent
Stood forth confess'd; for then the nation's soul
  Rous'd from its morbid dreams and lethargy,
No longer striving 'gainst Divine control,
  Echoed His fiat—" Make my people free;—
What you would share, grant all—the boon of
    liberty!"

Heir to a life eternal—fellow-heir,
  'Tis thus our Pilot would conduct us home;
'Tis thus He seeks to lead through faith and prayer,
  Unto the Father's house, whence we would roam;
When Gospel truth, when blessings fail to win
  The wayward child or nation that He loves,
'Mid Sinai's thunders, 'mid contention's din,
  These signal benedictions He removes;
And thus, through adverse storms, our frail depend-
    ence proves.

Then let us trust Him; howe'er dark the hour
  In which our trembling, fainting faith He tries;
Howe'er portentous be the clouds that lower
  Above our heads; the greater sacrifice

STRENGTH THROUGH ADVERSITY.

We yield to Him, the greater the reward;
And though to us His ways seem mystery,
And with our futile schemes but ill accord,
Let us take courage; well assured that He
Will grant us grace and strength through our adversity.

NOT RETURNED.

His regiment returns to-day, they told me so last night,
Who joy to welcome back again the vet'rans of the fight;
In accents hushed they made it known, the cause if you would learn,
His regiment returns to-day, but he does not return.

It seems to me but yesterday, so swift time's flight has been,
We trod life's pathway hand and hand, he ten and I fifteen;
He was my all; for ere those days there came a time of tears,
When death removed, from earthly scenes, our stay in earlier years.

And mother kissed her Gabriel, and father blessed
 his boy,
And bade me to protect through life our household
 pride and joy;
How swiftly he to manhood grew! How brightly
 shone that mind!
Brightly as only beam the souls so soon for Heaven
 designed.

My pride, my joy, my fondest hopes around him
 fondly clung—
God pardon if the homage due to Him the creature
 won!—
Then came to us and thousands more, another time
 of tears,
When ploughshares unto swords were turned, and
 pruning hooks to spears.

Men left the anvil and the loom, the homestead hearth
 and all
That rendered life most dear to them, to heed their
 country's call;
My idol stood among those men on that eventful
 day,
Dear as he was, and young in years, I would not bid
 him stay.

I buckled on his sword-belt, with a cold and nerve-
    less hand,
And saw him proudly march away, one of a valiant
    band;
Then turned me with an aching heart from that dread
    scene away,
Feeling that nought was left me now, save but to
    weep and pray.

Time passed; the war-cloud, rolling on, still dark,
    and darker grew;
Drenching our soil with precious blood of loyal, tried
    and true;
While he, unscathed as yet by harm, stood firmly at
    his post,
Vowing that he'd desert it not, whate'er might be the
    cost.

And I, how eagerly I read the news each battle gave,
Bringing my anxious cares to Him, whose power
    alone can save;
And then, as victory seemed more near, oh, how my
    spirit yearned
To welcome back my darling, when his regiment re
    turned.

That welcome I may never give; but in the future
  dim
My cherished one shall welcome me, when I shall go
  to him ;
The cause is known; the story sad I scarcely need to
  tell—
You'll learn it from the mournful words—at Wilder-
  ness he fell.

And stranger hands have buried him upon a stranger's soil—
In an unnoticed grave he sleeps, free from all earthly
  toil—
While deep into my throbbing heart these scathing
  words still burn—
His regiment returns to-day, but he does not return.

Sad record—one by millions borne—and millions yet
  to be,
Will ponder oft those records o'er in grateful sympathy ;
In sympathy for stricken hearts, that oft in secret
  yearn
To greet their war-slain patriots, that never more
  return.

OUR NATION'S GRIEF.

> "Oh, watch you well, by daylight,
> By daylight you may fear;
> But keep no watch in darkness,
> For angels then are near."

DAYLIGHT and darkness—How they mingle here,
  To soothe our grief, or mitigate our joy!
'Luring us onward toward that purer sphere
  Of hallowed bliss, unmixed with an alloy.
Daylight and darkness—They have come to us
  In all their force of brightness or of gloom;
Mingling the day-dawn's brilliant radiance
  With all the sombre shadows of the tomb.

Daylight—How flashed its fair, auroral star!
  Brighter and more resplendent burned its rays!
Though rendered lurid by the smoke of war,
  Men blessed its dawn and gave to God the praise.

That dawn was darkened by one cloud, alone;
  One only shadow did its glories wear—
Sorrow for cherished ones forever gone—
  And that, long since, we'd nerved ourselves to bear.

Then came the darkness—Ah, how swift it came!
  Like thunderbolt from cloudless zenith sped
The startling message—"Our loved Chieftain's slain!
  By an assassin's hand his blood was shed.
Rescued from murd'rous hands, our Premier lies,
  Maimed and disabled, on a bed of pain"—
Can Freedom still demand such sacrifice,
  Where human blood has deluged hill and plain?

"'Tis false!"—Thus argued Faith in tones sublime,
  While struggling Hope essayed her cause to plead—
"E'en Treason could not perpetrate such crime,"
  E'en Slavery's champions prompt so foul a deed.
Alas! alas! Our faith and hope, how vain!
  Once more the fluid o'er the wires is sped,
And anxious, breathless millions hear again
  The mournful tidings—"Our loved Chieftain's dead!"

Upon that signal morn the sun arose,
  In gorgeous splendor, like some monarch proud;
Struggled a while his glories to disclose,
  Then veiled his face behind each weeping cloud.
And why was this? 'Twas Nature's sympathy!
  Her pity for the aching hearts that bled;
Her sorrow for that untold agony—
  A nation mourning for her martyred dead.

Dead? Dare we say it? When, from ages past,
  An echoing voice resounds from shore to shore—
Though Error, thwarted thus, would shrink aghast,
  Eternal Truth shall live forevermore!
Eternal Truth none have the power to slay!
  He lives and reigns e'en in a world like this!
Where base Iscariots heartlessly betray
  Their Lord and Master with a traitor kiss.

Men thought they slew Him, when, by Jewish law
  Scourged before Pilate, He condemned stood;
When from the foot of Calvary they saw
  The last death agony, the crimson flood.
Men thought they slew Him in that horrid scene
  Enacted on Virginia's scaffold high,
When Harper's Ferry's hero hung between
  The snow-enshrouded earth and vaulted sky.

OUR NATION'S GRIEF. 243

Men thought they slew Him at our capital,
  Where glaring lights and dazzling scenes did blend;
And sympathizing hundreds gazed appalled,
  Yearning to save, yet powerless to defend.
But vain their efforts all! That Power Divine,
  Triumphant evermore o'er all His foes,
When crushed the casket which that Power enshrined,
  Has, Phœnix-like, from out its ashes rose.

Then, while we mourn, as nation never mourn'd,
  The fate of one in whom we've learn'd to trust,
Whose soul has passed beyond the mystic bourne,
  Whose dust now mingles with its kindred dust,
Let this blest thought our drooping spirits cheer,
  And to those spirits consolation give—
Though he has closed on earth his just career,
  In the good deeds he wrought he still doth live.

And if another martyr yet must fall
  To save our bleeding country, there was none
More ready to respond unto that call,
  More worthy to receive his God's "well done!"

OUR NATION'S GRIEF.

Ours is the loss, his th' eternal gain
    The bliss, enfranchised spirits know above;
For us the darkness—the sad funeral train;
    For him triumphant joy 'mid light and love.

Disposer of events, hear Thou our prayer!
    A suff'ring nation turns in tears to Thee!
Thou who dost deign the mourner's grief to share,
    Henceforth from blood-stain make that nation free!
May he whom Thy mysterious Providence
    Has made our leader in this signal hour,
As firmly lean on Thy Omnipotence,
    As him we mourn, when threat'ning clouds shall lower!

Chasten'd, but not dishearten'd we have grown,
    Feeling that, but for this sad tragedy,
Our nation's history had never known
    The crowning point of its sublimity.
Thus, of that nation's worth a conscious pride
    Is strangely mingling with the tears we shed—
Through keenest suff'ring we are purified—
    Peace to the memory of our righteous dead!

IMMORTALS.

Immortals! Who are they?
The 'franchised beings of the Spirit land?
  Or those who, cumbered with their cumbrous clay,
Still in probation tread this nether sphere,
Or, alternating between hope and fear,
  On its eternal confines waiting stand?

  Aye, all of these! I'd dare
Not to oppose the doctrines of philosopher or sage
  Who cope the subtle dogmas of Voltaire;
Who, to o'erthrow the creeds such dogmas wrought,
Their untired efforts to the contest brought,
  In deeds recorded upon history's page.

  I'd not presume to give
The flutt'ring, struggling, clay-imprisoned soul,
  A surer evidence that it shall live
In the hereafter, than itself hath known,
When, mindful of its weakness, at the throne
  It seeks for strength to reach its destined goal.

For he who e'er hath felt
The calm impress that spirit doth receive
  In such communion, or hath ever dwelt
Upon its earnest strivings for the right,
Its aspirations for unclouded light,
  Knows of that life, and, knowing, must believe.

Mine is a different task;
To point to those beyond the mystic tide,
  Whose untold glories, hidden by the mask
Of envy, prejudice, obscurity,
Dreamed not of thanks from millions yet to be,
  While in the martyr's ranks they nobly died.

Or those who yet in life
Tread humbly their allotted pathway here;
  Or, calmly gazing on the useless strife
For fame and power, seek but themselves to know
The duties God apportions them below,
  And to perform them, faithful, without fear.

Rome had her heroes; Greece,
Assyria, Carthage, Sparta, all had theirs;
  The olden world, whether in war or peace.

Boasts her immortals—spirits brave and bright—
Making the onward course of truth and right
   The constant burden of their ceaseless prayers.

   Peace, honor to their dust!
Not rightfully alone belong to these
   My poor laudations; they are held in trust
Within their native climes; where voices raise
And grateful hearts accord to giving praise
   In swelling pæans far beyond the seas.

   Columbia, my own
Belov'd country, turn I unto thee;
   Proud of my birth-right; proud that I have known
A heritage beneath thy skies; can claim
A sisterhood with those whose constant aim
   Was virtue—freemen, whom truth made free.

   Columbia! With thy
Name come memories of one, born
   Long ago beneath Italia's sky;
To whose great spirit there had been revealed
A mighty scheme; doomed long to be concealed,
   Ere it in glory hailed its triumph morn.

For eighteen years he sought
For recognition; waited, hoped, and prayed;
 Then came an answer; such as to him brought
Means meager, but such means as seemed to him
A welcome beacon, howsoever dim,
 Cheering him onward by the light it shed.

 Then followed fame, success,
Hatred, reproach, and e'en the dungeon-cell,
 For then, as now, the noblest souls claimed less
Of earthly homage than the baser kind;
To such, the impartial future has assigned
 Proud monuments that shall their goodness tell.

 It was not his to see
The friendly Banian planted on the strand
 He well might call his own; nor yet the tree—
The deadly Upas—by that Banian's side,
Diffusing, in an ever-flowing tide,
 Its fatal poison upon every hand.

 It was not his on earth
To mark that startling scene, nor those
 Which followed; nor to know the worth,

Of each convulsion ; but if clayless souls,
Foreseeing all things from their sinless goals,
   Know well the meaning of such fearful throes,

Then let us hope that his
Has shared with us the sorrow and the joy,
   The danger and the triumph; for his bliss
Must sure be purer near the " great white throne,"
If through this conflict he hath seen and known
   All of the triumph, free from doubt's alloy.

The noble spirits reared
Upon his soil for the great contest stern—
   Unmoved, unwavering, as that contest neared,
Some but with spiritual weapons armed—
Others with carnal—calm and unalarmed,
   Though hate's red fires around their pathway burn.

And as the war-cloud lowered,
The mighty revolutions that it wrought—
   The world's pet heroes sunk to craven cowards—
Her chosen cravens raised to heroes true,
Proving, as nearer their great triumph drew,
   Full worthy of the cause for which they fought.

But more I need not tell
Of those whom freedom ever shall revere;
  How nobly in her sacred cause they fell;
Some leaving honored names on fame's bright scroll;
Others whose records she may ne'er enroll,
  Immortal in the hearts that loved them here.

Nor yet that other scene—
The dazzling brightness followed by deep gloom;
  When he, our Chief—our modern Nazarene—
In the proud acme of his glory fell,
A martyr to the truth he loved so well,
  To fill henceforth a nation-rev'renc'd tomb.

Oh, 'twas a sight sublime—
The sorrowing millions in that funeral train—
  The dusky millions who'll revere, through time,
The deathless name of him who cared for them—
The brightest jewels in his diadem
  The tears they shed o'er their deliverer slain.

We who have, side by side,
Marked the fierce strife of darkness with the light,
  And light's eventual triumph—what just pride

We thus have shared; when, mingling oft our tears
O'er our immortals—fallen in those years
   Of gloom and terror—sacrificed to right.

In minor points we may
Agree to differ; but in this we should—
   We must united stand for aye!
Freedom demands it—spirits of our slain
Bind us together in one rendless chain—
   One common bond, cemented by their blood!

And of the laurels green,
That one by one have twined around the brow
   Of her, our mother country—none more bright
     shall be,
Than those which shall thereon ere long appear,
With the proud monuments which she shall rear
   To her immortals and to liberty.

Then let them, let them rise!
To be henceforth a sacred Mecca shrine
   To our successors; and as their young eyes
Gaze on them, let them teach to them the truth
That life is nought—nought e'en to buoyant youth
   When duty's call bids us that life resign.

And we who still survive—
To whom this glorious work seems but begun—
   In honor to our dead, let us e'er strive
All truth to raise, all error to subdue,
Claiming alike for ever grade and hue,
   Social and civil rights till victory's won.

All help is from on high;
And in the scales of justice no false weight
   Ere yet was found—then, though we sigh
Each day o'er wavering trust in human power,
So prone to fail us in some signal hour
   'Twill teach this lesson—God alone is great.

May He whose hand Divine
Has led us through this labyrinthian wild
   Thus far in safety, aid us to resign
Each grievous error for the common good—
Granting a nation, cleansed by human blood,
   A lasting peace—all pure and undefiled.

OUR ENSIGN.

"O Flag, beloved in better years,
  O Flag, baptized in blood and tears,
  O Flag, more sacred for your cost,
  We love you better for our lost.'

HERE, beneath the oak tree sitting,
  Gaze I on the distant town;
Gaze I on the varied landscape
  From the hill-side sloping down,
Clad in drapery of em'rald,
  Crimson, gold, and oaken brown,
'Neath yon vaulting arch of ether,
  Wearing its autumnal crown.

Sluggishly the Appomattox
  Winds along its destined way;
Glimmering in the effulgence
  Of the royal "king of day;"

Or reflecting from its surface
    Cloudlets, floating far away—
Golden clouds, and clouds of purple,
    Leaden clouds, and ashen gray.

Gracefully beneath yon tree-tops
    Mark our country's ensign wave!
Proudly proff'ring its protection
    To the loyal, true and brave;
Flutt'ring there as others flutter
    Over many a martyr's grave;
Bearing far aloft the colors
    Of the land they died to save.

Mingled shades of white and crimson,
    Shades of azure, glowing bright
Over all its heaven-hued surface
    With its stars of silvery white;
Truth and purity combining,
    Emblem of the might with right,
Emblem of the good, the holy,
    Blood-redeemed from error's blight.

And I think, while thus I'm gazing—
    Flag of freedom, floating free—
Musing sadly on the suff'rings
    Of the hosts that died for thee,

What such sacrifice availeth?
  When, throughout our land, we see
Evil's allies, plotting blindly
  'Gainst the cause of liberty.

And my spirit breathes a prayer
  For the good, the pure, the true;
For the triumph, aye and ever,
  Of the red, the white, the blue;
For its all-impartial shelter
  Unto every grade and hue;
Unto sons whose sable fathers
  In its own defence were true.

And as daily here I'm toiling
  'Mid a long-degraded band,
'Mid a race as dark and dusky
  As the hosts on India's strand,
Brought by cruel force amongst us,
  From their distant father-land,
Oft I query—when will justice
  Come to them from God's right hand?

Patience, soul! That prayer's answer
  Follows duly in the train
Of truth's triumphs; faithful, hopeful,
  Breathe that prayer once again!

Justice, mercy, peace, and freedom,
    For their cause was Jesus slain—
Christ doth reign, and since He reigneth,
    All He loveth, too, shall reign.

Farmville, Va., October, 1867.

GATHERED TO HIS FATHERS.

"There is no flock however watched and tended,
  But one dead lamb is there;
There is no fireside, howsoe'er defended,
  But hath one vacant chair."—*H. W. Longfellow.*

PICTURES within the realms of thought
  Are traced by memory's hand;
And vividly their scenes are wrought
  With talismanic wand.

Most prominent among them now,
  Upon the canvass glow,
Two scenes it was my lot to view,
  Not yet twelve months ago.

The first of these, an "old arm-chair,"
  Fill'd by an aged form,
That oft had sway'd amid the winds
  Of life's relentless storm.

A face with kindly smile for all,
    A head of silvery hair;
While voices full of childish mirth,
    Mingle their cadence there.

They cluster 'round the " old arm-chair,"
    They climb the envied knee;
Impatient each fond kiss to share,
    In innocence and glee

* * * * * * * *

The scene has changed—the snowy shroud,
    The coffin and the bier,
'Mid solemn, sad funereal rites,
    Successively appear.

Vacant now stands the old arm-chair,
    While childhood seeks, in vain,
For th' endeared form 'twill ne'er
    On earth behold again.

A grassy grave near a rural grove,
    Where zephyrs gently sigh;
And a name upon a plain white stone,
    Meets the gaze of the passer-by;

Is all that remains of that ripen'd shock,
  The Father hath gather'd home;
Safe from each chilling blast that blows,
  Each tempest that yet may come.

These warlike times were not for him;
  For his was a life of love;
And he fled these bloody scenes below,
  For more peaceful scenes above.

Then let him rest near that rural grove,
  Where the zephyrs gently sigh;
And his loved name on the plain white stone,
  Meets the gaze of the passer-by.

For the passer-by who knew him best,
  When this earthly sphere he trod,
Could but read in that name—"An honest man
  Is the noblest work of God."

ONE YEAR IN THE SPIRIT-LAND.

WRITTEN ON THE FIRST ANNIVERSARY OF THE DEATH OF A FRIEND.

One year in the spirit-land,
  The land of the pure and fair;
One year on the star-gemmed strand,
  'Mid the bright-winged seraphs there;
One year by the crystal fount
  That flows from the throne of God;
One year near the holy mount
  Only by angels trod;
One year in the golden streets
  Of that perfect and sinless sphere,
Hast thou revelled 'mid heavenly sweets,
  While I have been toiling here.

Tell me, enfranchised soul,
  In celestial bliss secure,
Art thou at thy shining goal
  Becoming each day more pure?

When my spirit, from earth-cares flown,
    Seeks thine in those regions fair,
Shall each by the other be known,
    And loved as 'mid worldly care?
Or hast thou, through bewildering joys,
    So advanced on thy heavenly way,
That I, amid earthly cloys,
    May not hope for that rapturous day?

To my mental ear doth come
    A reply;—It is thine, I ween,
Though I in pure regions roam,
    And thou in a world of sin;
In that future, auspicious hour,
    When thou from that world art free,
The unfailing, all-cleansing Power
    Thy spirit shall guide to me:"
Father, " thy will be done!"
    That fainting spirit saith;
Till that shining goal be won
    Strengthen my hope and faith.

GOING TO THE SPRINGS.

Dust, dust fills the air like a vapor,
   In the highways of fashion and trade;
And the mercury, ranging toward blood-heat
   By Fahrenheit, stands in the shade.
Trunks, valises, band-boxes, portmanteaus,
   Are pack'd till they almost o'erflow;
And the Cowperthwaites, Courtneys, and Chestons,
   Are in haste toward the wharves seen to go.
"Whither now?" cries a 'wilder'd spectator—
   "What is it this retinue brings,
Thus crowding our wharves and our steamboats?"
   'Tis responded—"They're going to the Springs!

"To the Springs, to be crowded and jostled,
   And tortur'd by Fashion's restraint?
To compete with each other in flirting,
   Or who can most gracefully faint?
To the Springs to be stung by mosquitoes
   At night, and by gnats through the day?

GOING TO THE SPRINGS.

To the Springs, where for each inconvenience
    You're expected to handsomely pay?
Why not seek at once some quaint farm-house,
    Whose quiet rusticity brings
Untrammell'd, the comforts you're needing?
    'Twould be cheaper than going to the Springs."

"Aye, there is the rub," my good fellow,
    Such comforts, we very well know,
Can always be had for a trifle;
    But 'tis there all the common folks go.
The Mudlarks, the Popham's and Drewsters,
    Can seek such resorts when they please;
Would you dare to insult us by making
    Us equal to people like these?
No! rather each costly annoyance
    Let us have! Though our money has wings,
While it lasts, we must keep up appearance,
    And persist still in going to the Springs.

There are heart-aches in yon spacious mansion;
    There are debts by its inmates unpaid;
There are battles, hard battles with fortune,
    Through dread of yet being betray'd.
Too poor to compete with rich neighbors,
    Too proud to acknowledge defeat,

Defrauding the honest of payments
  They're always unable to meet,
They are sinfully, madly pursuing
  A course that remorse ever brings;
And, too cowardly to brave an exposure,
  Are recklessly going to the Springs.

Did you hear that loud laugh of defiance?
  Did you mark that still beauteous face?
Still beauteous; though dire Dissipation
  Has left there his ruinous trace.
She is the lost child of a bankrupt,
  Once left without money or home;
A victim of false education,
  On the broad road of ruin to roam;
Despising all honest employment,
  Or the peaceful reward that it brings,
She is foil'd in the snares of the Tempter,
  And recklessly going to the Springs.

Thus, thus upon Life's dusty highway,
  The victims of folly and pride,
By hundreds and thousands are thronging,
  Regardless of what shall betide.
Whenever we yield thus to Fashion,
  And sacrifice all to appear

GOING TO THE SPRINGS.

On a par with aristocrat neighbors,
   A cringer to favor and fear,
We daily and hourly are treading
   A path that disaster e'er brings;
And like Cowperthwaites, Courtneys, and Chestons
   Are foolishly going to the Springs.

Dupes, dupes of aristocrat folly
   Are thronging our nation's highway;
Each year they've grown stronger and stronger,
   Each year have extended their sway.
In vain has Democracy striven
   That rule and that sway to restrain;
Those haughty aristocrats, ever
   Have scorn'd from that sway to refrain.
To the brink of disaster and ruin,
   They have borne us on swift-sailing wings;—
Alas, how this brave Yankee nation
   Has sadly been going to the Springs!

Alas, for the victims of fashion!
   The victims of folly and pride!
The dupes of aristocrat folly,
   That throng us on every side!
God shield both the people and nation,
   That thus must be ruled by their sway!

Grant them vict'ry in striving for freedom,
  Make them conquerors now and for aye!
Redeem them from ev'ry disaster,
  And ev'ry dark sorrow she brings!
And restrain them henceforward from yielding
  To recklessly going to the Springs!

EARTH'S GREAT ONES.

"The drying of a single tear
Hath more honor, fame, than shedding of seas of gore."

Who are earth's great ones?—are they those whose sabre,
  Hath spilled the life-blood of their fellow-man?
Who to the sound of fife and drum, or tabor,
  March bold and fearless to the battle's van?
Say, were *they* great, the firm, undaunted hero,
  The fearless conq'ror of each realm and State—
Ambitious Bonaparte, the tyrant, Nero?
  These were the champions whom the world calls great!

Time-honor'd Washington, renown'd Pulaski,
  France's noble son—immortal Lafayette;
Those who now foremost stand 'mid Truth's great war-cry—
  These, these are names we may not soon forget.

But, turn aside—turn from the scroll of glory—
    Go trace each by-path in the realm of Fate;
There pause awhile, and read each simple story—
    The hidden annals of th' unknown great.

Go linger thou beside the dying pillow,
    And mark that gentle one who kneels in prayer!
Or by yon urn beneath the drooping willow,
    List to her words of comfort spoken there!
Go scan each haunt of vice, each gloomy prison;
    Talk to the crime-stained wand'rer of his fate;
And, when from error's chains he hath arisen,
    He'll bless the kindness of the unknown great.

Go to some home, howe'er obscure and lowly,
    To where the sister, daughter, mother, wife,
Doth oft exert an influence most holy,
    To snatch the wayward from the snares of life.
Such are earth's great ones; those unknown in story,
    Whose names ne'er stand upon the list of fame;
But, who amid the brighter realms of glory,
    Eternal, blest inheritance shall claim.

THE SIGHING OF THE PINES.

THE snow-flakes lie in stainless drifts upon Virginia soil—
A soil impov'rish'd by the tread of ill-paid sons of toil;
Of swarthy sons whose Saxon sires their masters strove to be,
Till War's loud clarion, echoing far proclaim'd that they were free.
I'm thinking of that triumph now, and as the day declines,
I list with hushèd spirit to the sighing of the pines.

What ails you—bright green visitants 'mid Winter's icy reign—
Ye em'rald pledges 'mid his snows that spring shall come again?

Yours seems a cheerful mission—a mission grand
and high—
Fair emblems of unchanging bliss, then wherefore
do ye sigh?
Why over valley, hill and dale, as the bright day
declines,
Falls on my ear your smothered wail, ye softly
sighing pines?

I know that darkest crimes have been enacted 'neath
your shade,
And warriors in their gory graves beneath your
branches laid;
But rather be your strains henceforth to joyous
numbers strung—
Joyous because of all the good forth from the evil
sprung;
Then as each sadly sighing sound its mournful air
resigns,
I'll with more pleasure list to you, ye softly sighing
pines.

Ye heed me not! Your sighings still fall sadly on
my ear—
Sadly as o'er a lov'd one's grave doth fall affection's
tear;

THE SIGHING OF THE PINES. 271

Yet gentle is your gravest note; and when the
 weary soul
Seeks refuge from the ills of flesh at its appointed
 goal;
And weeping friends to mother earth its clayey
 house consigns,
'Twere sweet to rest beneath the shade of softly
 sighing pines.

Farmville, Va., New Year, 1868.

IT IS FINISHED.

"When Jesus, therefore, had received the vinegar, he said, 'It is finished!' and he bowed his head, and gave up the ghost."—*John* xix. 30.

"It is finished! It is finished!"
   Was the agonizing cry
Heard amid appalling darkness
   On the Mount of Calvary.
Finished? Yes! For our salvation
   The sufficient, perfect plan—
Finished all the tribulation
   Felt and known by Christ, the man.
But beyond that earthquake—darkness—
   Midnight gloom 'mid blaze of day—
In the realms of light and glory,
   Christ the Sov'reign lives for aye.
And, unfetter'd by the thraldom,
   The incarnate One endured,
His eternal Power and Godhead
   Reign e'erlasting has secured.

IT IS FINISHED.

"It is finished!" says the mourner,
    Bending o'er the lowly bed,
Where, in weary hours departed,
    She has sooth'd the aching head.
Whisper'd words of consolation,
    To relieve each painful throe,
Ere the damps of the "dark valley,"
    Settled on that pallid brow.
Yes, 'tis finished! ev'ry sorrow,
    Ev'ry earthly toil and strife;
Ev'ry trial and temptation
    That besets the path of life;
But, unto the soul immortal,
    Saved by th' atoning One,
In the realms of light and glory,
    Life eternal has begun.

"It is finished!" says the student,
    As he twines around his brow
Wreaths of th' unfading laurel—
    "Finished is the conflict now!
Ev'ry obstacle I've conquer'd,
    Ev'ry battle I have won;
And I leave these halls of learning,
    Conscious that my work is done."

IT IS FINISHED.

Is it thus, aspiring student?
  Is thy toil forever o'er?
And, will Duty's voice, commanding,
  Point to labor nevermore?
No! for many moral combats
  In the "bivouac of life,"
Yet await thee—to the warfare!
  Gird thy armor for the strife!

It is finished! it is finished!
  Language ever breathed in vain!
For each conquest in Life's battle
  Bids us other trophies gain.
Nature everywhere proclaims it!
  In the earth, the sea, the sky!
Action, progress are her watchwords—
  Watchwords for Eternity.
And the poet speaketh truly,
  When, to mortal man he saith,
In an unmistaken language,
  Fraught with wisdom, hope, and faith—
"Onward, onward, onward ever,
  Human progress none can stay;
All who make the vain endeavor,

www.ingramcontent.com/pod-product-compliance
Lightning Source LLC
Chambersburg PA
CBHW031948230426
43672CB00010B/2092